For

Fawziya

Women Who Want More

How to Create a Balanced and Fulfilled Life

Dr. Rana Al-Falaki

Published by Richter Publishing LLC www.richterpublishing.com

Book Cover Design: Richter Publishing images by www.123rf.com

Editors: Margarita Martinez

Book Formatting: Monica San Nicolas

ISBN: 978-1-945812-91-0 Paperback

DISCLAIMER

This book is designed to provide information on self-improvement only. This information is provided and sold with the knowledge that the publisher and author do not offer any legal or medical advice. In the case of a need for any such expertise consult with the appropriate professional. This book does not contain all information available on the subject. This book has not been created to be specific to any individual people or organization's situation or needs. Reasonable efforts have been made to make this book as accurate as possible. However, there may be typographical and or content errors. Therefore, this book should serve only as a general guide. This book contains information that might be dated or erroneous and is intended only to educate and entertain. The author and publisher shall have no liability or responsibility to any person or entity regarding any loss or damage incurred, or alleged to have incurred, directly or indirectly, by the information contained in this book or as a result of anyone acting or failing to act upon the information in this book. You hereby agree never to sue and to hold the author and publisher harmless from any and all claims arising out of the information contained in this book. You hereby agree to be bound by this disclaimer, covenant not to sue and release. You may return this book within the guaranteed time period for a full refund. In the interest of full disclosure, this book may contain affiliate links that might pay the author or publisher a commission upon any purchase from the company. While the author and publisher take no responsibility for any virus or technical issues that could be caused by such links, the business practices of these companies and/or the performance of any product or service, the author or publisher have used the product or service and make a recommendation in good faith based on that experience. All characters appearing in this work are fictional. Any resemblance to other real persons, living or dead, is purely coincidental. The opinions and stories in this book are the views of the authors and not those of the publisher.

CONTENTS

THANKS AND ACKNOWLEDGMENTS

I have wanted to write a book for years. Whenever I voiced this, I'd be asked what it would be about. I could never quite answer that other than to know that everything I have experienced in my life could be used to inspire others. Having created enough space, all has finally aligned and made this possible. However, we are never alone, and I certainly could not have done this on my own. I owe so many people huge thanks.

Firstly, thank you to my mother Fawziya, to whom I dedicate this book. She has been the greatest inspiration in my life as a powerful, determined, luminous, loving woman. While she died over 20 years ago, she remains with me, continually championing me on. Thank you to my father, Dhia, who believes in me wholeheartedly, inspires me, has had to play the roles of both father and mother, and has done it so effortlessly and well. Thank you for keeping me afloat in the difficult times, and riding the waves with me when I keep on pushing and striving on to further adventures. Thank you for being my anchor and reminding me I can do anything. Thank you to my children who are equally as proud of me as I am of them, and who have had to put up with me being holed up in my office, but never complained. Thank you to my partner who always has my back and doesn't laugh at me when I run into the woods to hug trees, as I did when I completed my first draft. Thank you to all my friends and family for your unwavering belief and support. It means so much.

The more conscious we become, the more we surround ourselves with people who are like us. I feel so blessed to have finally found my tribe, and am so grateful to each and every one of you for the roles you have played in my being able to produce this book. I'd write an entire book of thanks if I listed you all by name, but will give a special mention to Anna Bokova, my coach, and to Leanne Wild and Bridgette Simmonds, my trainers and mentors, who also led me to my wonderful publisher. Thank you to Alice Northrop, my creative creator, for all her help and ideas, and of course to my dear friend Diyari Adbah for his support, inspiration and belief in me. Thank you to John Eggen for his mentorship and authenticity, and to Christy Tryhus, my book coach extraordinaire, who pushed and supported and guided and laughed with me. Thank you of course to Margarita, my editor, the whole team at Richter Publishing, and of course Tara herself, who is truly a guiding light.

And lastly, but certainly not least,

Thank You, Universe!

PRAISE FOR THE AUTHOR

I felt Rana's empowering presence from the day we met and it grew over time through her genuine interest in others, empathy and understanding, warmth and authenticity. It's an absolute delight to know a rare woman like Rana.

Anna Bokova
Executive Director, Global Transaction Banking
First Abu Dhabi Bank

Rana stands out. She has a presence that is magnetic. She's brilliant, funny, charming, determined ... the list goes on. We met as colleagues and we ended up becoming friends. As colleagues I saw Rana as extremely hardworking, present, and focused. She was always willing to help and give that extra little bit of support. As we became friends I learned more about her personally, and I'm in awe of how she transmuted the challenges in her life into personal power and success. She really is one of the most inspiring people I've met. When I am in her presence I feel uplifted, encouraged, and supported. I am so excited for her next steps and can't wait to see where life will take her.

Aarti Inamdar MScBMC
Digital Art Director
Florida, USA

Rana is an inspiration! She's a compassionate and highly intuitive coach. She's driven to achieve success both in her personal life and for her clients. After just one coaching session I gained valuable new insights and my whole perspective changed, which has had a big impact in my life. I wish her every success.

Wendy Parrott
Administrator for Youth Cancer Trust
United Kingdom

Rana coached me during the last stage of my training to become a coach. She helped me during this transition by tapping into my values, beliefs, and blocks that were preventing me from reaching my goals. She was very precise to find the questions I needed to resolve my doubts and she has a great energy when coaching. Working with Rana has been a pleasure.

Marita Aldana Sanchez
Executive Assistant, Phillips, and Coach
The Netherlands

Rana's an awesome coach, with deeply intuitive insights. She is Deep. Gifted. Insightful. Strong. Powerful. A truly beautiful person ... a truly gifted and impactful coach; a real breath of fresh air, with such powerful intuition. Rana's such an inspiration and continues to inspire everyone she meets.

Ugochi Bede
Head of Talent
Nigeria

Rana has always excelled in every aspect of her diverse background due to her fantastic work ethic, enthusiasm, and compassion. Her knowledge together with intuition places her in the perfect position to inspire and help others to achieve their goals, both personally and professionally.

Peri Mehmed
Dental Surgeon
United Kingdom

I have known Rana for many years, as a colleague and most of all as a dear friend. In that time I have experienced many challenging situations and Rana has always guided me through. I am so pleased she has finally written a book to inspire others to achieve their goals.

As a woman she is confident, with an amazing work ethic and drive. She has a presence that lights up a room when she walks in. She has a vast knowledge in her field and a true perception and understanding of life.

Lesley Walton
Practice Manager and Payroll Director
United Kingdom

I had just moved to the UK when I met Rana. From the day we met I felt a deep connection. I felt overcome by this amazing energy. And as we talked, I felt relaxed, and so confident! Everything became so easy to understand and the world made sense in a positive way. It was like there were no more clouds in the sky, only sunshine. I feel I don't struggle so much, but when I do, in a simple talk, Rana just shows me the way to become even more positive and I just feel relaxed.

The confidence she gave me allowed me to now pursue a new career and be a new woman, with a new future. I know that I have the ability to achieve it all!

Patricia Viveiros
Psychologist, Childcare
Portugal and United Kingdom

The minute I met Rana, I was in awe of her calmness, nurturing, and caring nature. She has an ability to make everyone she meets feel like they're the most important person in the room and takes a genuine interest in them and their lives, instantly putting them at ease. She doesn't ever judge; she completely understands the complexities of people's lives and the turmoil of life. She always offers an empathetic shoulder or ear and offers an alternative, unbiased view of the scenario.

Rana has an aptitude for seeing greatness in people when they don't see it themselves. Rana is the most extraordinary leader. Her unwavering support is always in existence despite what is going on in her life and this is something I will always cherish and hold so dear.

She is an inspiration to so many, including myself. We need more people like Rana in the world to make it a more loving, peaceful place.

Keelie Greaves
Business Owner
United Kingdom

Rana has this innate ability to know what I am thinking before I even articulate it myself, as if she can almost read my mind. She has an ability to empathize and connect with you that instantly makes you feel better and more understood and you leave the conversation feeling more empowered.

Rana has always been and continues to be so very hardworking and driven and tuned in to whoever she is talking to and that ability is truly inspiring.

It is a privilege to know her.

Gita Sharma
Dental Surgeon
United Kingdom

FOREWORD

Dr. Rana Al-Falaki has dedicated her career and life to helping others in the most professional and genuine way. Her talks are inspirational, and her personality is larger than life. Anyone who has had the pleasure and privilege to listen to her can testify to the fact that she is truly an amazing and genuine human being with a kind heart and doesn't withhold anything.

When I met Rana for the first time, I felt like I had known her all my life. A true friendship and mutual respect were felt straight away. I also sensed that we were both from the same breed; the breed that dedicates their life and energy to helping others and to create a better today for a better tomorrow for all.

We both started in the business of caring about and for others, and in my experience, as a health professional and a life and business coach, we meet a lot of people who could benefit from our insight and help. I find the ones who serve the longest and in the most genuine way are the ones who pour their soul and their entire life into it and peel themselves layer by layer, regardless of how hard or painful that might be, in order to help others.

You see—you cannot help anyone and be honest with anyone if you can't be honest and transparent with yourself.

While we both still enjoy a successful professional career, one of the most important lessons we have both learned over the years is that true success is not in having more money or more fame and power, but rather in human dignity and helping others enrich their lives.

I remember a few years ago I was shooting a documentary in central Mexico. We were helping to build schools in remote parts of central Mexico so that kids could have better access to education, instead of traveling for miles and endangering their lives getting to a remote school. During my stay I learned a big lesson: it is all about human dignity. Some of the kids and the workers had absolutely no means to secure their future. They lived from one day's hope to another, but despite that, they were very proud and always smiling. They were just so happy to be part of this amazing task in improving the lives of children. They had so much love to give. Most of the helpers lived well below the poverty line, but they were mighty and powerful and noble in that they were contributing to the world becoming a better place. It was all about human dignity, and staying true to your core. The documentary went on to win an Emmy Award.

Every aspect of life is full of surprises, from amazing and joyful moments to problems and issues that may seem beyond the scope of repair or resolution. Life is about challenges and obstacles as much as great and happy moments; that is why it is 'Life,' and to be able to make sense of everything around us can be overwhelming and paralyzing sometimes. Therefore, to help find insight and make sense of most things that life throws at us, it is important to have a true and genuine voice who is willing to share their own experience and insight to help others move forward instead of standing still and feeling helpless.

Everyone is charged with immense energy, but during times of need and when we are most desperate, not everyone is equipped with enough knowledge to redistribute and redirect that energy in the right direction to help turn situations around. By introducing the uniqueness of core-energy™ coaching in this powerful book, Rana shares her expertise in showing how to shift that energy to make us feel and do better in life, creating a life of abundance, health, and happiness both professionally and personally.

Rana's ability to make sense of complex matters—clearing the fog—and making them simple to grasp, is unique and she is truly gifted in that respect, doing it so well in this book.

Rana has the ability to listen with her entire body; she listens with her ears, her eyes, and her entire body language reassures you that she is fully with you, and feels you entirely. She is there in that moment in life, in this universe, with you, and it seems like she doesn't want to be anywhere else but where she is, giving you her attention, which is why I think she is so amazing and such a unique human being. Somehow, she manages to give you the same feeling as you read this book—like she is right there with you, championing you on.

I have had the privilege of listening to Rana and every time I listen to her, I feel she adds value to our lives and this world can be a better place because of her. I am proud to call her my friend and she is someone I have huge respect and admiration for. And in my opinion, one should take every opportunity to listen to her and read her book over and over again and take every opportunity to learn from her programs.

This world is a better place because of people like Rana Al-Falaki. She has shared with me that her mission and her passion in life is to empower others to be their true selves, to shine, to feel fulfillment and joy. I truly believe that this book delivers that and so much more.

Dr. Diyari Abdah, MBA
Best-selling Author of *The Winning Way* (co-authored with Brian Tracy) and *Success 360*, Ziglar Legacy Performance Coach, Executive Producer of the Emmy-Award-winning humanitarian documentary *Armonia*, Cosmetic Dentist, and Adj. Professor

INTRODUCTION

If you are reading this book, then the chances are you want more from your life. There may be something missing. You may know what that thing is, but be unsure how to get it. Or you may not even know what it is but still feel stuck in some way, perhaps restless, perhaps unfulfilled, perhaps feeling that there has to be more to life. You might be feeling out of balance in some aspects of your life, or repeating patterns that just don't seem to get you anywhere. That is certainly a description of me some years ago. I wished at the time that someone could help me, but had no idea where to turn. People and books could give me insights, but then I didn't know what to do with those insights. I struggled and wished someone could wave a magic wand and give me what I wanted, which essentially was a feeling of freedom, peace, purpose, joy, abundance, and complete fulfilment. That is what my inspiration for writing this book has been—to help you get whatever it is you want in a faster, easier way than my own journey.

I was born in London in the early '70s to immigrant Arab parents. As the youngest of three, I was nicknamed the 'accident,' but was reassured by my parents that I was the best accident that could have happened! My life seemed to progress uneventfully, growing up in the middle-class suburbs, going to an all-girls school, then off to university to study dentistry. I excelled academically and socially, with lots of friends and rarely a 'B' grade in sight! It was when I hit my twenties that I truly lost sight of myself. Memories of childhood abuse came flooding back to me after being blocked out. I developed an eating disorder. My relationships never worked out quite the way I hoped and I experienced emotional abuse and broke off two engagements in that decade. Most significantly, my mother, who was so much more than a best friend, died of cancer. I was left home alone. My brother and sister both left to live with their partners and my father fled the country, no longer able to cope. All the while, I continued to do incredibly well socially and professionally, becoming one of the country's youngest specialists. No one was party to my inner turmoil.

I was delighted to turn 30—it was a new beginning! I met my husband, who surely must be different because *I* was different. We had three beautiful, healthy children and the perfect house. I had my own highly successful clinic and was widely sought after professionally. What people saw was the happy, engaging woman smiling at patients. What they didn't see was that she was doing that while having miscarriages— five in total—or that her milk had come in after she'd just given birth to a dead baby and gone back to work the next day. What people saw was the busy, wonderful mother and career woman who was beautiful and slim. They didn't see the inner turmoil she had in trying to hold her marriage together and keep her husband happy, never feeling that anything she did was good enough for him, and feeling completely powerless to change it.

By the time I turned 40, my career was skyrocketing. My business was thriving. I was becoming world-renowned for my pioneering work, I was healthy, and so were the people around me. Surely life could settle down now and I could finally be happy. How unfair would life be if I had more tragedies? Hadn't I suffered enough?! Well, I went through a divorce; my sister got cancer and didn't want treatment; my career (my only salvation in the past) suddenly threatened to come crashing down;

I got myself into yet another emotionally abusive relationship; and then I was diagnosed with a chronic health condition.

You couldn't write about that! Only that is exactly what I am doing, because after all that, I found what I had been looking for all these decades. I found joy, fulfillment, a way to balance. I found my inner power, and I now have a deep need in me to help anyone who wants to do the same.

I was a periodontist, a dentist who specializes in treating gum diseases, for 20 years. These are chronic diseases that not only impact the mouth, but also affect the whole body and have psychological impacts. A great deal of my time was spent not only performing surgery on patients, but getting to know them. I had to tap into their mindset in order to help them change their behaviors—to quit smoking, reduce stress, eat healthily, lose weight, spend time on themselves, and take ownership of their condition. I also taught and lectured widely all around the world, pioneering more patient-friendly treatments. My passion is teaching and helping people. In fact, it is even more than that— it is empowering people.

Having shared my story with you, I'm sure you can understand that just helping people in a medical capacity was no longer enough for me. If I could find and have what I wanted in life, it felt like my purpose was to help others have it too, so they didn't have to suffer the way I did or take quite as long to find it. I needed to move that help beyond the scope of just health and medicine into people themselves, into their core. I trained as a core-energy™ coach and you'll hear me refer to that throughout this book. The idea of core-energy™ coaching is to connect your outer goals—your desires, the things you want—to your inner core; the thing that makes you, you. This very powerful process helps people to enjoy rapid, long-term, extraordinary results.

In this book I take the process a step further by explaining the relevance of not only the need for energy and enthusiasm and how you can achieve that, but also the importance of balancing that energy in all aspects of your life. If you have both energy and perfect balance in all aspects of your life, then you have it all. *All* being everything you could ever wish for.

Wherever you are on your journey, this book can help you.

Now, I appreciate that we all have very busy lives, and if you'd asked me a few years ago to take time out to read a book while I was juggling a million and one other things, I might have laughed in your face. Or I might have bought the book you recommended and then left it to gather dust on the bookshelf until I was ready.

If, however, you are ready to take the next step and discover how to create a balanced, fulfilled, and energetic life, I invite you in.

In the first three chapters, I'll teach you strategies that you can apply to every aspect of your life, starting with the first big step of defining what it is you actually want. I'll introduce you to the concept of energy, how that shows up in our lives, and discuss how to set boundaries.

In chapters 4 through 10, we'll tackle every aspect of your life. In writing this book as a busy woman myself, I have written it *for* busy women. I have tackled the most common problems that affect us and explain what we can do to solve them. I'll delve deeper into issues that affect your work life, relationships, families, dietary concerns and body image, health, financial status, fun, and time-management challenges.

At the end of each chapter there are exercises to help develop your learning and insight. I have left space for you to write down answers and thoughts, but some may prefer to have a notepad handy, or a device to record thoughts and answers. I have also made worksheets for most of the exercises available to download for free from my website www.lightchangescoaching.com. Complete the exercises in your own time, without pressure to complete them on anyone's schedule but your own.

Also on the website, you will find an audio recording of a centering exercise. This is a useful daily practice and only takes five minutes. Additionally, you will find some guided meditations that I refer to in the chapters which are free to download, as well as other resources to further heighten your learning.

In the final chapter, I'll bring it all together for you and we'll talk about what the next steps in your journey might be.

For now, sit back, relax, buckle up, and enjoy the ride!

CHAPTER 1

KNOWING WHAT YOU WANT
"I CAN'T!" – YES, YOU CAN!!!

"... people don't know what they are striving for. They waste themselves in senseless thrashing around for the sake of a handful of goods and die without realizing their spiritual wealth."
~ Aleksandr Solzhenitsyn

It won't surprise you to know that most of us don't know what we want. We think we do, but when asked the question, can't quite articulate it. However, most of us know what we *don't* want, and if you start to ask people I can bet you that will be their first response. How can something that is so incredibly simple actually be so hard? It gets harder as we age, and I'll share the reason with you.

Can you remember when you were a child and someone asked you what you wanted to be when you grew up? The answer might have been a nurse, a hairdresser, an astronaut, or in my case, a teacher. Of course, nowadays, kids might reply with, "A You-Tuber!" There's a common theme going on here: as children, we mold ourselves to our surroundings whether it's our parents, teachers, TV shows, or the games and toys we play with. Not only that, but at that stage we're still too young to have been affected by negative self-beliefs, the most prominent one being—I CAN'T. We also haven't yet been in this world long enough to be affected by energy influencers and limiting beliefs, which I'll talk about later. Ask any child under the age of five what they want to be when they grow up, and aside from the initial typical shyness and shoulder shrug, you'll probably get a really cute answer. And why the hell shouldn't it be?

So what changes? Life happens. Beliefs are inflicted on us as children. Other people's values and fears become embedded in us, and it's only by working on ourselves as adults, becoming conscious, and taking the time to get to know ourselves, that we start to adopt our own beliefs and values, our own influencers, make our own choices, and step into who we truly are in order to know what we truly want, rather than what other people want for us.

Let me give you an example. Let's talk about money. Money is often a big taboo, and we'll go into it in a lot more detail in a later chapter. But for now, take a moment to think about what your parents told you when you were growing up. Did you hear phrases like "money doesn't grow on trees," "we can't afford that," "oh, that's so expensive," "we don't have enough," "it's rude to talk about money," or anything else along those lines? Now think of your own attitudes towards money today. Do you use similar terms or have similar thoughts? Do you actually want more money, but feel too embarrassed to voice that desire out loud? I can think of multiple clients of mine who fall into that category. It's no surprise, when I question them deeper, to find that they recall those phrases from their past and realize they chose to take on those beliefs as their own, albeit unconsciously. It comes as no surprise that once they are aware of it and in a position to make a more conscious choice, they realize they can actually choose to think something different. I'll teach you how to do exactly the same thing.

Just sticking with money for a minute—I remember shortly after I got married in my early thirties. When I was a child, my father's business was hit by the '90s recession and so my mother was the main money-earner, working three jobs to get us through school and maintain a household. Not surprisingly, given that history, to me £100 (which you can think of as the equivalent to $100) was a *lot* of money. But the strangest thing was I would hear my husband talking about things costing *"only"* £100, and what a bargain he thought that was! Listening to him talk like that, and knowing that we had a mortgage and bills to pay, I was appalled by what I viewed as his wasteful spending because we had totally different views on the subject, with mine certainly being a result of my upbringing. At that time in my life, I had not yet chosen to adopt my own beliefs. Would I have been embarrassed back then to voice out loud that I wanted more money? Oh my goodness, yes!

So, back to the subject of knowing what you want. The reality is you do actually know, but the answer is stored somewhere inside of you, locked away and buried so deep under piles of fears or limiting beliefs which have come from your experiences that you can't quite hear it. But it's knocking, trying to find a way out into the open. And when you hear that little voice whispering to you, "What is it you want?", you need to be ready to answer.

KNOCK DOWN THE FENCES SO YOU CAN SEE

This is an exercise that on the surface seems so simple, but as you do it, keep giving yourself permission to truly go all out and play, allowing yourself to just think big, with no holds barred.

When I do this exercise with clients, I keep reminding them that they have to step out of the box of restrictions and limitations in life as they know it now. To give you an example of what I mean: if I were to ask you what job you want and you have children, you might not allow yourself to think about the true job you want because you are limiting yourself by your current reality where you need to only work during school hours because you have no one to help you. If I were to ask you what an adventurous life might look like to you, and deep down you want to climb Mount Kilimanjaro, you might not voice that because you have an arthritic knee or suffer from chronic fatigue syndrome or fibromyalgia, and therefore limit your choices according to the current reality that is your physical state as you know it.

Hopefully you get the idea, and so the only rule for this exercise is:

There are no rules!

Allow yourself to be free!

Don't let the BUTs into your process!

Don't worry about the HOWs!

No one else is listening except YOU, so there's nothing to be ashamed of.

I understand that there will be some things beyond your control such as an ill parent, for example, so please try to set those aside for the purpose of allowing yourself to dream. I'm not saying forget such things or negating their importance, and we'll discuss later in the book how you can feel better and more in control of those kinds of situations.

The questions for this exercise are listed here, but if you'd like the worksheet, or want to listen to the guided meditation, download them for free at www.lightchangescoaching.com.

I'd like you to imagine that there are no limits. You have all the money you could ever wish for—however many millions or billions that may be. You have perfect health; you are oozing with enthusiasm and energy. There's no one telling you what you can and can't do; there are no one else's feelings to consider in your choices other than your own. You have plenty of time each day to fit everything in; you are in control of your own life.

Now I'd like you to consider each aspect of your life in turn and think about the answers to some of the following questions as they apply to you. Jot them down, always keeping in mind that here, there are no limits.

Relationships – Intimate

a) What do you want in a relationship?

b) What does your perfect partner look like?

c) What are you doing together?

d) How are you communicating?

e) How are you showing up as part of that partnership?

f) How is your partner supporting you and vice versa?

g) What do you do for fun together?

h) What is the single most important thing you need from your partner?

Relationships – Social

a)   What is your social life like?

b)   How many friends do you have?

c)   How well do they understand you?

d)   How do you want to be able to feel and behave around your friends?

e)   How do you support your friends?

f)   How do they support you?

g)   How often do you see them?

h)   How do you communicate?

i)   How do you enjoy your time together?

j)   What do you and your friends do together?

Relationships – Family (children and/or parents)

a)   What does your family life look like?

b)   How are you feeling and acting in your family environment?

c)   How are you supported?

d)   Where are you living?

e)   What do you do together?

f)   How do you feel at the end of a perfect day together?

Health and Aging

a)   What does it feel like to be in perfect health?

b)   What does your body look and feel like?

c)   What does your skin look like?

d)   How much energy do you have?

e)   How much are you laughing?

f)   What can you physically do?

g)   What can you mentally do?

h)   What are you eating?

i)   How do you feel when you wake up in the morning?

Money

a)   What kind of home do you have?

b)   What does your bank account look like?

c)   What kind of holidays are you taking?

d)   What kind of car are you driving?

e)   What gadgets and luxuries do you own?

f)   How are you using your money to help others?

Fun and Enjoyment

a)   What are you doing for fun?

b)   What adventures are you experiencing?

c)   How much are you laughing?

d)   What brings you the most enjoyment?

e)   What do you love doing?

Career and Lifestyle

a)   What are you doing for work/during the day?

b)   How does it feel to wake in the morning and look forward to the day?

c)   How many people do you engage with?

d)   How active are you?

e)   How much fun are you having?

f)   How are you feeling at the end of the day?

g)   How are you portraying yourself to others?

h)   How appreciated are you?

i)   How much variety do you need?

j)   What do you love most?

Personal Development and Spiritual Awareness

a)   How are you relaxing?

b)   How are you growing and learning?

c)   How much are you trusting your intuition?

d)   How are you engaging in creativity?

e)   How much are you honoring your values?

f)   How does it feel to be free of fear?

g)   How does it feel to trust?

h)   How much balance is there in your life?

i)   What ritual or practice might you be engaging in?

Even if you only managed to answer a few of these questions—CONGRATULATIONS! It's a great start and I'd invite you to revisit this exercise again once you reach the end of the book and truly step into your power. We'll be going into each of these areas in more detail in the following chapters, but for now, I bet you're thinking, "Okay, so this is what I want, but what do I have to do to get it all?" Well, those are precisely the secrets I'm going to be sharing with you in this book.

Before we move on, I just want to touch on a few things I mentioned earlier: limiting beliefs and energy influencers. A limiting belief is any thought that limits us in some way from achieving our goals or desires. As I've already discussed, we adopt these beliefs from what other people tell us as we're growing up, from our environment, our friends and partners, the media, and what we read. To give you an example, the news is full of tragedies and disasters. If you were to watch the news on a daily basis, you'd probably be filled with fear that the world is an ugly, violent place and believe that there is nothing but conflict. Now, if we take that to the next level, depending on your past, this belief could have different degrees of power over you. Say you were subjected to abuse as a child, and then hear a news story about a child being abused by a man. (Please excuse the stereotyping here—it's only a generic example.) Hearing that may evoke a reactionary emotional response in you and consolidate your belief that all men are abusers. In turn, that may add to your lack of engagement with men in your adult life, or inability to enjoy a healthy relationship.

Conversely, someone with no personal experience of the same may have feelings for the victim in the story but be more blasé and simply saddened by the issue, rather than being so affected. I might add here that I stopped watching the news years ago because it did nothing other than fill me with fear and depress me. Why waste your time being subjected to other people's fears? We have enough of our own to deal with! That s of course, just my opinion.

Let's take another example—the classic issue of an upbringing where you were led to believe that 'you can do anything, be anything, succeed at anything in life,' versus the voice of 'you'll never be able to do that—you're not talented enough; you're not pretty enough; you're not slim enough; you're not clever enough.' While the first person is more likely to grow up daring and adventurous and willing to push boundaries, the latter may grow up carrying such baggage potentially into every aspect of their life, not being daring enough to ever try due to the power that this limiting belief has on them. The classic emotion these beliefs evoke is one of insecurity and is known as "the gremlin" inside us. In coaching people, I aim to tease out these limiting beliefs and guide you to feel powerful enough to choose new beliefs that will serve you so much better.

As well as limiting beliefs, the other aspect that can impact whether we achieve what we want is energy influencers. Think of how you feel when you wake up in the morning, having made a plan to go to the gym, but then can't follow through. What was it that stopped you? Was it that you couldn't be bothered? Did you wake up feeling slimmer than you thought you would and so the motivation was gone? Did something better come along? Was your head or another part of your body hurting? Were you aware of how much else you also had to get done that morning and so maybe your headspace wasn't in the right place? Did no one in your family support you in making working out a priority? Was it too cold to get out of bed? Or anything else? Whatever it was, that limiting belief had an influence on your willingness to engage and execute the plan—on your energetic engagement.

These energy influencers come in six categories: spiritual, mental, emotional, physical, social, and environmental. This is something for you to consider when you find yourself unable to complete a task. As a core-energy™ coach, I measure your energy levels as they relate to specific goals and aim to unblock the barriers to your being able to achieve them. The exercises in this book will help you in that process. You can read more about this at www.lightchangescoaching.com.

Now let's get back to helping you learn how you truly can have that dream life you just wished for!

CHAPTER 2

WHY CHOOSE THE HARD WAY?
LET ME HELP YOU CHOOSE AN EASIER PATH

"Possessing material comforts in no way guarantees happiness. Only spiritual wealth can bring true true happiness."
~ Konosuke Matsushita

I could use this opportunity to tell you my entire life story in more detail, at which point it might either pull on your heartstrings, or you'd end up thinking, yes, that's fine, but what about me, and how does that relate to what I need to know? It's a little bit like when we're growing up; our parents tell us that they know better than us, purely based on their life experiences. Then, of course, we pick and choose from what they say and frequently learn the hard way, much to the frustration of our parents, who then relish the ability to say, "I told you so!"

This all effectively links into one common theme: people won't do anything they're told to do unless it truly resonates with them in some way.

Think of a classic example of someone who is a smoker. No matter how many times people tell them they should stop, providing all the reasons, unless that person really wants to and makes the decision, it's not going to happen. My coaching clients often tell me that one of the things they really love by the end of our sessions is the fact that they themselves have chosen the actions that they need to take, which in turn gives them the power. The fact that it came from them rather than from me telling them what to do helps propel them into true action, which leads to much more sustainable long-term results. So in other words, this is a very long way of saying that I'm not going to tell you my life story and based on that, tell you what to do, but I *will* give you some pointers that I think might help you reach that perfect, joyful balance faster than I did.

I'm sure if someone had been there to take me under their wing and guide me in these particular philosophies, I might not have gone down such difficult paths in my life and experienced quite so much pain. Of course, the pain I experienced has made me who and what I am today and allows me to now be able to write this book and share my learnings to help you.

There are three key points that we need to address, but first I'd like to introduce you to the concept of energy, which is a common theme for all of them.

As things occur in our lives which we do not ever truly deal with, this creates a kind of sludge in our bodies. Think of starting off with a great big hole in the ground. Each time we do something wrong and apologize, but never really deal with the problem, or each time a particular event happens in our lives and we end up feeling hurt but don't take the time to stop, reflect, and clear the air before moving on, it's like pouring mud into the hole. At the start, the mud might be quite light, so you can negotiate your way through it if you put on a pair of wellies and just start wading. But as the mud gets more and more solidly packed, it takes harder work and stronger legs to try to get through.

In the end, we're so exhausted that we can't reach the other side of the hole because our legs just don't have the energy to take the next step. Or the boot gets stuck in the mud and your foot comes out, which means there's a part of you missing that then stops you from progressing any further.

Now I'd like you to try to think of the body in the same kind of way. Every time we don't deal with things, it's like our body gets filled up with sludge and so the energy that needs to flow within our bodies is suddenly unable to. Think about how blood flows through our arteries, capillaries, and veins. If one of those vessels happens to get a little bit clogged up, the blood might find another pathway through. But eventually if everything gets blocked up, you may end up having a heart attack or stroke.

Similarly, we also have channels that carry energy through our bodies. Each time we don't deal with something emotional in our lives, one of those channels starts to get a little bit blocked up, and so the energy may need to find another way through, or it may simply take longer to pass through that particular channel. In other words, we start to get slowed down and then, the more baggage we take on without clearing the blockage, the harder it is for the energy to flow through. We slow down and slow down and eventually something comes off or goes missing, like that muddy boot. In other words, we stop functioning very well.

This reduced function may not seem obvious to start with. It may simply mean that you're more tired when you get up in the morning or you find yourself not quite as motivated to exercise or are not as clear-thinking at work. Gradually you may start to notice it in different forms such as back pain or frozen shoulders or headaches. This can then progress to chronic diseases such as diabetes and heart disease, gum disease, high blood pressure, or illnesses like chronic fatigue syndrome and fibromyalgia.

Let's talk a bit more about energy.

I'd like to take this opportunity to explain a little bit more about energy so that you don't think it's some kind of bizarre form of alternative medicine that doesn't relate to you. When we eat food, it works its way down to our stomach and into our small intestine. Following digestion, the nutrients are distributed throughout the rest of our body and into our cells. We have all these little things called mitochondrion in every single one of our cells, which use those nutrients, metabolize them, and thereby create energy. Of course, if we don't eat enough, then our energy levels are low and we feel weak. Think of the phrase "I've used up all my energy reserves" after completing a tough workout or pushing yourself to the limit in some other way.

Think of a moment when you got really worked up about something, whether it was a fight or a fright. Once that confrontation or fear was over, you suddenly felt really deflated and exhausted because you expended most of your energy reserves. So energy is there all the time, flowing through and around our bodies.

You've probably heard the terms "good" and "bad" energy used. People talk about someone or something as having a "good vibe." _Vibe_ is an abbreviation for _vibration_, meaning a vibration of energy. In truth, there is no good or bad energy, and each type of energy has its uses in appropriate circumstances. You'll hear me referring throughout this book to two particular types of energy and to energy levels, which are the levels of energy we resonate at and are the vibes we are giving off at a particular time.

The following concepts contain my interpretation of the copyrighted work of Bruce D. Schneider and the Institute for Professional Excellence in Coaching (iPEC), including the seven levels of energy that I refer to throughout this book.

Catabolic energy encompasses levels 1 and 2. To help you relate to this, think of the word "catalyst," which is something that triggers a breakdown or catastrophe. Catabolic energy is a draining, destructive energy, and is the type that releases cortisol and adrenaline into our bodies, which are the markers of stress. We repel success when we vibrate at this level.

Anabolic energy (think of anabolic steroids used to build muscle), is a constructive, building, healing energy. It releases feel-good chemicals such as endorphins into our bodies. We attract success with this type of energy vibration. These are levels 3 through to 7.

I will refer to them throughout this book to illustrate the effect they have on our lives. Studies have shown that the greater our levels of anabolic energy, the greater success, happiness, and fulfillment we experience in life. This forms the fundamentals of core-energy™ coaching. For more details about this and what each of the energy levels represents, visit www.lightchangescoaching.com. I have outlined the basics of each energy level below as I will refer to them throughout the book.

	Core Thought	Core Emotion	Core Action/ Result
Level 1	Victim	Apathy	Lethargy
Level 2	Conflict	Anger	Defiance
Level 3	Responsibility	Forgiveness	Cooperation
Level 4	Concern	Compassion	Service
Level 5	Reconciliation	Peace	Acceptance
Level 6	Synthesis	Joy	Wisdom
Level 7	Non-Judgment	Absolute Passion	Creation

The other thing to bear in mind about energy is that it can't be created or destroyed. It can only be transformed from one form to the next. The most effective way of allowing it to flow through us is by clearing the sludge.

I mentioned at the start of this chapter that there are three particular areas to address when it comes to creating an easier path in life, or a path through the 'sludge' as it were.

Forgiveness

The first aspect involves forgiveness. Back when we were kids on the playground, if we accidentally knocked someone over, teachers told us that we needed to apologize. As children, we automatically assume saying "sorry" means that we are forgiven and it's all forgotten about. In actual fact, this subject goes an awful lot deeper.

When I was 12 years old, I was repeatedly sexually abused by my grandfather over about a two-year period. So traumatic was the event that I actually blocked it out until I was in my early twenties and it all came flooding back to me. The obvious thing seems to be the need to forgive my grandfather, which I did shortly before he died in his late nineties a few years ago. The last time I saw him he asked me to forgive him, obviously knowing that he was soon to be heading to the grave. Really though, it's so much more complicated than that. I didn't only need to forgive my grandfather, but I also needed to forgive myself.

For years, I blamed myself for allowing it to happen the first time. Then I blamed myself for allowing it to happen repeatedly. And I blamed myself for being stupid enough not to tell anybody at the time. Sure— any counselor or therapist could say to me, "But here was a man who you loved so much and who was threatening to kill himself if you told anybody. So how on earth could you as a young teenager take on the responsibility for the death of somebody you loved? It's no wonder that your emotions were confused to say the least."

But that's a little bit like saying "yes, I really know I should stop smoking." In other words, had I undergone such counseling, my thoughts at the time would probably have been "yes, I know what you're saying, but it's not really connecting with me" because I was the one who had to make the conscious choice to truly let go and forgive myself.

So once I forgave my grandfather and myself, you'd think that the energy channels would be a little bit clearer, but no, it doesn't end there. I managed to find my voice and tell my mother about what had happened. Of course, she was completely devastated about the fact her father could do such a thing and was incredibly confused about her own feelings. Did she stand up and make it public in our family? Or confront her father about it? No, she didn't. I went along with this, but it became apparent over time that both she and the situation were something I needed to forgive. Admittedly, at the time, I wasn't in a state where I could really talk about the details of what had happened and I was concerned about my mother's feelings.

I suggested my mother might want to speak to her sister about it. I wanted my aunt to know in order to ensure that the same thing didn't happen to her daughter. That discussion did apparently take place, but unfortunately things also happened to her daughter. My mother then died a year later, before we'd ever really had a chance to talk about it any further because I had continued to bury it, and that required more forgiveness of myself. I also needed to forgive my aunt for allowing things to happen to her daughter. Now, being from an Arabic family, this thing really did get buried because you can't have public humiliation going on. So even though this man had done something so terribly wrong, people couldn't know because of the shame that it would bring on the family. My aunt didn't want to share it with her husband because she thought, unlike her, he would probably go absolutely crazy and take some kind of vengeance on her father. I needed to forgive society.

A few years later, I also told my father. You can imagine that 12-year-old girl desperately wanted her father to take a stance and shout out that this kind of behavior was not okay and defend her. That didn't happen. He replied, "Oh well, you know, he's a really sick man. He must be mentally ill." So I also needed to forgive my father. That didn't happen until a few years ago when I was in my forties.

I also told my brother and sister, but when we'd go visit our family in Bahrain, I would see them still being the dutiful grandchildren, greeting my grandfather, kissing him on both cheeks, sitting at his table, and spending time in his house. In feeling this incredible betrayal and isolation from my siblings and the rest of my family, you can start to understand how forgiveness is not straightforward. It was only in my forties that I confronted my brother a little bit more about how I felt at the time. He replied, "I never actually realized it was that bad because you'd never been as graphic in telling me what had happened."

Well, to me that isn't really an excuse, but that aside, once I had my say and expressed my expectations and feelings and forgave everybody, I finally felt able to breathe because I'd cleared the air. It was like this massive release of energy that had been holding me back. I was finally able to move truly forward in my life, on every level, which is something I'll touch on when I talk to you about relationships in later chapters.

Let's look at another example. One of my clients couldn't stop herself from eating lots of sweet and fatty foods once she started. She tried to compartmentalize by saying that she was having an indulgent weekend with her girlfriends, so she would give herself permission to do that and expect to cut down again once she hit the weekdays, but compounded with that was an enormous sense of guilt and frustration and to some degree, self-hatred. Yet she couldn't stop herself and just kept on repeating the same cycle. She exercised, and got herself a personal trainer and a nutritional coach, but still couldn't consistently deal with her attitude towards food. It was only when we started to explore deeper that we learned there was much more to the story that she needed to release but hadn't realized.

Her mother had put her on repeated diets. Her father had made comments about how round her face looked and how it wasn't anywhere near as pretty when she was overweight. There were cultural issues to do with people commenting on her weight whenever she went back home to visit relatives. No matter how much her husband told her she was beautiful and that he loved her just the way she was, my client wasn't able to love herself. Rather than hearing what he was saying, she was still hearing those voices from her childhood.

It was only when we exposed those memories in our coaching sessions that she realized there was a lot of forgiving to do. She had to forgive her parents, her relatives, her culture, and herself in order to release the hatred and the emotions that emerged after she ate those kinds of foods. Once she made those discoveries and we put actions into place to bring about a more permanent behavioral change, then that energy was released and she was able to progress forward.

I hope by giving you these two examples, you realize that forgiveness is not as straightforward as saying "sorry" and then someone else turning around and saying, "That's okay." Events from our past are often deeply rooted and it's in that forgiveness of ourselves and others that we start to learn to truly love ourselves. There is the classic line of, if we don't love ourselves, how can we expect anyone else to do the same? But it's so true.

So I challenge you to think of what there is to forgive in your life. What might have happened in your past relationships? You might be able to identify particular patterns that give you clues to the need for forgiveness in those areas of your life. It might be like my client— something to do with health and body image, or it might be a situation you're currently in with your career or home life where you can't seem to move forward. That's really the key: an inability to make any significant progress because you're stuck. You're stuck in the mud, and the next step you take is going to leave the boot in the mud, and a part of you behind.

EXERCISE PATH TO FORGIVENESS

The first key is to actually recognize that there is an issue that needs to be dealt with. You might choose to hire a coach to help you identify the problem. Or you could start with personal exercises such as learning to love yourself.

1-   Loving Your Reflection

Stand in front of a mirror and truly look at yourself for five minutes a day, whispering, "I love you. I love you. I love you."

Initially you might notice the messy hair, the blemishes, or wrinkles. As you carry on looking, your consciousness goes deeper and deeper, and the image that you see will start to change and can turn into something much more emotional if you really engage in the exercise. Try doing it consistently for at least a week. It's always a great idea to keep a journal and note down what you see during the exercise. As you go deeper, you will start to engage with the more meditative state and things may really come up for you.

2-   The Four Phrases

I heard this one from Joe Vitale in his book, *The Secret to Attracting Money, a Practical Spiritual System for Abundance and Prosperity*. I'll call it the Four Phrases. He describes some research done by somebody who went into a hospital and meditated with patients using four phrases. Strangely enough, an awful lot of the patients started to get better. These four phrases are incredibly powerful. Take just a few minutes a day to say them to yourself, either quietly in your head or even more powerfully, out loud. The phrases are:

I am sorry.

Please forgive me.

Thank you.

I love you!

You might want to think about a particular subject. So if we take the food issue and beating yourself up about the fact that you've just had a massive slice of chocolate fudge cake, you might then say, "I'm sorry," thinking that you're sorry for the fact that you hated yourself for doing that. Then ask for forgiveness. Then be grateful for being forgiven and express love to yourself, which is the most powerful thing you can have, and truly the key to everything.

So this is a great, really simple exercise that you can adopt into your everyday life. I find myself doing it if I have chosen not to go to the gym one day and feel incredibly guilty about it and have tried to rationalize all the reasons why it didn't happen. The energy of guilt doesn't serve us; it just drains us. So I'll apologize to myself, ask for forgiveness, be grateful for that forgiveness, and remind myself how I do love myself. I'll repeat it to myself about 10 times for a few minutes. And the energy release is exceptional. It feels like my mother giving me a huge warm hug and making me feel like everything is okay.

3- Who Needs Forgiving?

Start to explore any issues that you have in your life and create a plan to deal with anybody who may have had an influence in a particular area of your life, and who may need forgiving along with you. Like I said, hiring a coach who can help you with that deeper exploration is often a great idea.

Gratitude

Gratitude can help you wade through the mud a hell of a lot faster and get unstuck. If we go back to childhood once more, we were taught to say thank you for everything. I'm a stickler for that with my kids. If I put their food in front of them, I expect a thank you. If we go out to a restaurant, I expect them to say thank you to the waiter. If they are given a gift, I certainly expect to hear thank you. And after we've had a great day out together, it fills my heart when my kids spontaneously thank me. It's not so much that I've given them anything material, but that they're expressing their gratitude for having had fun quality time.

I feel very proud to have polite children. But what does expressing that gratitude do for them and what can it do for you? Let me share a typical day in my previous life as Dr Rana Al-Falaki, periodontist. Patients who came to me had chronic diseases and had often been experiencing something truly debilitating in their lives, which included the inability to eat comfortably, feeling self-conscious about their smile or bad breath, perhaps waking up with blood on their pillow, being unable to function comfortably in a social environment, and generally feeling quite unwell. So what on earth did they have to be grateful for? When I met a new patient we'd go deeply into their history and see if there'd been any stress in their life. Though I've touched on the reasons for that as it relates to energy, there are also a great many scientific explanations for how stress affects the immune system and leads to chronic illness, including gum disease.

After hearing a patient's complaints, they might then go on to tell me the stressful time they were having with their elderly parents and teenage children. Or they'd say how they were going through menopause, so their moods were really erratic and they were putting on a lot of weight. Or they were arguing with their partner and had a really horrible boss at work who didn't have any faith in them and was so controlling. Or their sister-in-law had just died, leaving young children behind, and their brother was devastated and had also just been diagnosed with cancer. Or it may have all happened to just one person! You can imagine how, not only would my patients be in floods of tears, but I, too! And that was before I'd even done the dental exam!

What on earth would somebody with that kind of life story have to be grateful for? Has life ever seemed like a downward spiral where one thing happens and you focus on how tragic that was? And then the next thing happens and the next. In the UK we tend to joke, saying these things are like buses—nothing for a while, and then everything all at once; such is the beauty of London transport.

Instead of focusing on all the tragedies in life, my patient, let's call her Betty for the purposes of this story, could also have said, "I'm grateful to my dentist for referring me to you because I know you're going to be able to help me. I'm grateful for the fact the sun is shining outside today. I'm grateful because I've got two legs to walk on. I'm grateful for the fact that we have money and can pay our mortgage. I'm grateful for the fact that my children and partner are healthy. I'm grateful for the fact that I have friends."

Naturally, Betty's mindset would have been in no mood to look for that gratitude. However, gratitude is also a little bit like buses; the more we focus on it, the more we have the potential to find more and more things to be grateful for. In expressing that gratitude, our energy lifts and we release the sludge that's inside us. In the end we become so practiced at it that we just keep seeing things to be grateful for all the time and the things that were controlling us somehow don't have quite as much significance and are then no longer as debilitating. Being consistently grateful gradually shifts what you see from focusing on the negative to focusing on the positive, focusing on what you *do* have rather than what you *don't*, focusing on what you *do want* rather than what you *don't want*. In focusing on opportunities rather than challenges, expressing gratitude raises your energy levels and allows you to refocus on feelings of love. Betty was resonating too much in Level 1 victim mode to recognize that finding something to be grateful for could have truly helped her.

In my own life, when I see the rain pouring down, I don't say, "Oh, it's such a miserable day." Instead I say, "I'm grateful for this rain because the flowers and trees are happy to receive water. I don't have to water them, and my garden will look lovely." Do you see how I managed to put a positive spin on it?

So how can you incorporate gratitude into your everyday life?

We are all busy, so I truly believe in starting off small and then building your way up. I'm a big fan of multitasking. I wake up in the morning and the minute I go into the shower I'm thinking about all the things that I'm grateful for. Toothbrushing, shower, *and* expressing gratitude, all within five minutes!

I wake up in the morning and think:

- o   I'm grateful for my health

- o   I'm grateful for my home

- o   I'm grateful for my three wonderful children.

- o   I'm grateful for the fantastic day that I'm going to have today

- o   I'm grateful for the weather outside

- o   I'm grateful for the peace and quiet

- o   I'm grateful for the people I'm going to be able to help today

- o   I'm grateful for the food I'm going to nourish my body with

- o   I'm grateful for the exercise that is going to energize me

- o   I'm grateful for the meditation that will allow me to connect to my higher self o   I'm grateful for my children's smiles when they see me in the morning and when I pick them up from school

o   I'm grateful for the time we will spend together this evening.

o   I'm grateful for peace and harmony

o   I'm grateful for the chance to express gratitude throughout the day.

You see, when you start looking for things to be grateful for, the list becomes endless.

It doesn't need to be the big things like the money in your bank account—it could actually be the things that touch us. And the more of those that we have, the more of them we see, and the more our energy lifts and we feel love.

Another thing that I get all my clients to do is to keep a journal by the bed. If you bury a journal away in a drawer, you can bet it's not going to get used. The journal sits by my bed and every night before I go to sleep, I make a point of picking up the journal and writing down a minimum of three things that I'm grateful for that day. Even if on the surface it seems to have been a horrific and stressful day, in just taking those few minutes to think about what there is to be grateful for, I inevitably find something and it clears my energy before I sleep. I've noticed that since I started expressing gratitude through a journal at night, not only do I get all the benefits we've talked about, but I also get a much better night's sleep by focusing on all the positive points rather than the worries and tragedies that may have affected my day.

It's great to try to get everybody at home involved in gratitude exercises. I have a big jar on our kitchen counter with a notepad. Every time someone passes that jar, they jot down something to be grateful for on one of those pieces of paper and pop it in the gratitude jar. By the time it's full, it looks like a jar of sweets. It's something the kids absolutely love doing and is a fun way that we've been able to get my kids to really focus on the good things in life rather than who picked on who in the playground.

You can look at expressing gratitude in so many different ways. I invite you to be as creative as you want, but really start to notice the shift that occurs when you've engaged in gratitude for as little as a week.

EXERCISE PATH TO GRATITUDE

1- Express everything you have to be grateful for with a sense of anticipation for the positive things to come in the day and consider doing this while multitasking, which might mean while working out, boiling the kettle, driving to work, or like me, while I'm brushing my teeth or in the shower.

2- Place a gratitude journal somewhere where you can see it and access it very quickly. Even if you prefer to journal in the morning, it's still a good idea to also write something in that gratitude journal just before you go to bed at night.

3- Set up a gratitude jar and make sure it's as visible as possible. Put paper and pen right next to it and have fun with it.

4- Have a gratitude fest! This is a great fun exercise you can do with other people where you set the timer for at least three minutes and tell someone all the things that you have to be grateful for. The first minute or two may be obvious things around you, but as you keep on going past two minutes, you'll find so many more small things. Just watch your energy shift in the smile that comes to your face. Watch your partner's face as well because I bet you that energy will be infused into them and they'll be smiling too, and then you can reverse roles. This is something I do with my kids every now and again, and if we happen to be on holiday when we're on top of a mountain or on a beach, we all start screaming out "thank you!" with our arms raised above us and shout out everything we have to be grateful for.

My kids think I'm a little bit crazy, but they love my crazy side.

Spirituality

I'd like to discuss a topic that can have a lot of stigma associated with it. Spirituality is not religion. For some people, it may mean the same thing. Others will question how they can be spiritual if they are atheist and don't believe in God at all. Of course, there is an overlap, but one's spirituality is really about one's connection to something or someone. If somebody believes in God, then understandably they feel connected to God and as if God is talking to them. Others use spirituality as a form of defining their religion (a religion of spiritualism), and you will often hear about them feeling connected to a source or the divine or light.

According to the *Oxford Dictionary*, 'spiritual' is defined as "relating to- or affecting the human spirit or soul as opposed to material or physical things. In other words, it is anything non tangible and most likely non measurable."

Now, you can imagine for someone like myself who's been a scientist for so many years, anything that is not measurable is deemed nonexistent since you can't conduct experiments on something intangible. However, even if you don't consider yourself to be spiritual, have you ever had a gut feeling about something? Or a sense of fulfillment and joy within you without knowing why? That is part of your spirituality. Part of what relates to you as the human spirit or soul.

Spirituality encompasses multiple aspects including:

- o   feeling connected to your purpose or something bigger

- o   your determination

- o   your commitment

- o   your fulfillment of desires

- o   your ability to create a life balance and perspective

- o   your faith and trust

- o   your confidence

- o   your resilience

- o   alignment with your values

- o   your goals and your vision

- o   having something to look forward to

Think of being really excited and looking forward to a holiday. The holiday is the tangible aspect that you're looking forward to, but also consider the feeling you're going to have when you're on holiday, which may be one of freedom, relaxation, fun, and enjoyment. None of that can be measured on a scale.

So spirituality really is about being your true self, living by your values, and aligning yourself with people and situations that are compatible with those values. Have you ever been in a relationship where you never felt completely comfortable? It might have been an acquaintance, a working relationship, or a more intimate one, but did it feel as if something was missing or uncomfortable? Well, that may well have been because you were in a relationship with somebody who didn't align with the same values as yourself. Have you ever felt like you're just drifting along doing things for the sake of it, without ever feeling fully engaged?

I often think of people who sit in tollbooths on the highway, taking money from each car as it passes by, all without any human interaction or chance to say thank you or have a chat and smile. They just take the money, press a button, take the money, press the button, take the money, press a button, and continue to do this for an eight-hour shift.

I look at these people and think, "Oh my goodness, what kind of purpose do they have?" And yet they seem to be functioning perfectly happily. Of course, that's just my opinion based on my perception. But one of those people in those booths may be looking at it in a completely different way. They may be thinking that they're taking the money and allowing somebody to pass through a barrier on the way to a great holiday. They may be seeing themselves as opening the gateway to people being able to get to work. They may be taking pride in the fact that they're helping to control traffic, being as efficient as possible so drivers don't get stressed. Or they may be thinking that they're playing a key role in a company that's earning money and which may also be reinvesting that money into better roads and giving to charity, for example. They may feel connected to a purpose. It just reinforces – who am I to judge?

Listening To Yourself

Another important aspect about spirituality is listening to yourself. What feels right for you? Going with those instincts certainly requires faith and trust in yourself. Some people think of it as listening to God; others listen to the divine or to a source or their higher self. For the purposes of this book, we'll talk about listening to your higher coach. That aspect of you that hasn't been affected by all the events in your life and wants to lead you on the path to fulfillment. It's there to give you a bit of advice every day.

Spirituality is also about being present, not in bodily form, but by truly paying attention. How many of us have heard our loved ones or children telling us a story while we've been washing the dishes and then turned around and simply agreed with what they said without having paid any attention whatsoever? That aspect of being present is not just with and for somebody else, but it's also about being present with ourselves.

This is where the concept of mindfulness comes in. Try to be mindful in everything you do. That might be with every step that you take toward your workplace—watching your feet move and thinking about that, rather than about the million and one things you have to do when you get to work or distracting yourself on your cell phone as you go. It might mean being mindful of the food that you eat and being present as you take every mouthful and chew and taste and swallow. When you're mindful about eating, it also gives you time for gratitude, which is another bonus. You actually end up eating less when you do it mindfully as your stomach has time to feel when it has had enough before you overstuff it. That's a great tip if you want to lose a bit of weight—yet another bonus to spirituality!

Spirituality is about making conscious choices, which means truly choosing to do something because it aligns with your values and beliefs and purpose, which comes back to being your true self. Think about the word enlightenment. *"I am enlightened."* Those with spiritual beliefs may understand that to mean that a source has filled them with light (energy), but just think about how we use that term on a daily basis. You can look at someone and say, "Wow, you're all lit up" as a means of commenting on the person being happy and excited. We might say, "You're glowing!" We haven't flicked a light switch and truly made them glow like a lightbulb (unless you're like my seven-year-old who loves to shine flashlights on you in the dark when he's supposed to be in bed asleep!), but they're lit up from within and the light is shining from the inside out.

Why is that person glowing? They might be feeling quite joyful. What made them feel joyful? It was probably a sense of fulfillment and happiness, which in turn was probably related to feeling driven and connected to a purpose. Then we come full circle to being connected with your higher self, your higher coach, Source, The Divine, God, or whatever and whoever you want to call it. We can take it a step further still. When someone asks to be enlightened, by saying, "Enlighten me!", we can proceed to explain ourselves or a situation to that person. And in so doing we are connecting with that person and sharing a part of ourselves. A part of our light. A part of our energy.

Think of the word "awaken." When we get up in the morning, we awaken from an unconscious state. We also use it as a term when we come out of some kind of trauma or have a sudden realization and say, "I woke up!" That may not mean we physically woke up and got out of bed. It just means we woke up and saw the situation differently through different eyes, through connected eyes, through aligning with our true self, with our values, thereby effectively stepping into our power. I always smile at the term my American friend used to frequently use when she wanted you to see things as they truly were: "Wake up and smell the coffee!" How true and apt that statement is.

So how can you do it? How can you relate to spirituality and understand what it means to you? How can you awaken to consciousness? How can you understand what your true self is and have the guts and determination to present yourself to the world in that way?

For some, it may take a huge tragedy in their life. You'll hear about people who thought life just couldn't get any worse, and yet it just kept beating them down and down and down until they woke up. They then used those opportunities to turn their life around. Some may need more than one attempt at awakening before they actually start listening. I was certainly one of those people. I've already shared with you that my mother died when I was in my early twenties and that was an opportunity for me to wake up and engage with my true self.

After my mother died, I had a chat with my roommate at university, who, being a fellow atheist, said to me, "You know that this is it, Rana.

She's gone and there is absolutely nothing more. That's it." I questioned long and hard, how could that possibly be it? Friends took me to see clairvoyants, so desperate was I to hope that my mother would speak to me through those people. I felt completely and utterly lost. I felt completely disconnected. I had no purpose, much as I desperately tried to find some reason for why my mother and best friend could possibly leave my life. I remember writing a poem called "My Anchor," which was basically about my mother and how I was completely lost at sea without it. Without her.

I had a chance to wake up at that point, but then buried it by finding other purposes in my life, like immersing myself in my studies and postgraduate training. I had another opportunity when I found myself in an incredibly emotionally abusive relationship in my late twenties. That relationship did actually have a wonderful purpose in that the person introduced me to authors such as Paolo Coelho, Deepak Chopra, Tony Buzan, and Eckhart Tolle, whose book *The Power of Now* had only just been published at the time. I emerged from that relationship completely broken, physically ill, with no strength, and completely lost other than having an incredibly successful career. Having been introduced to all these wonderful, profound readings, I had a chance to connect further. But once again, having gone through the trauma, the chance got buried, and I distracted myself with career success.

When I got married, my husband was an atheist and not at all impressed with my then much-stronger spiritual beliefs, so in trying to please him, rather than being myself, I completely buried all of that aspect of my life away. Even my books were hidden behind closed doors for fear of his ridicule and disapproval.

Each time something tragic happened in my life, I would once again have an opportunity to awaken and would briefly turn to what I called my spiritual guides and angels but never had the guts to follow through with my instincts. I never really listened to myself or adopted anything as a daily practice. I suffered five miscarriages including giving birth to a little boy at 20 weeks. I was immensely unhappy during parts of my marriage, doubting myself as a person and felt so incredibly alone. Thankfully, I was also truly blessed with three beautiful children.

Following my divorce and the loss of several friends as is often the case in such situations, I then had to contend with the thought that my sister was headed to the grave, the same way that my mother died with a diagnosis of aggressive breast cancer.

Every relationship that I had, whether intimate or work-related, seemed to have some degree of abuse, some sense of feeling trapped and unable to make choices, of being held back and not being allowed to fly, of never truly being seen. But was it that I was not seeing, or more to the point, that I was not really showing my true self?

It was only in 2017, in my forties, following yet more emotionally abusive relationships and a chronic illness, that I finally woke up for good. I shed the shackles of a successful business that wasn't quite fulfilling me anymore. I shed the patterns of abusive relationships and along with that, I let go of chronic illness, fatigue, an eating disorder, and a lifelong debilitating relationship with food. I finally said to the world, "This is me!" Not just the woman who had been an incredibly successful clinician, researcher, university lecturer, public speaker, trainer, and business owner, but this is *me*: a woman who truly deserves to be happy and loved, who is a wonderful mother, whose purpose in life is to help people, who is healthy and vibrant and isn't going to accept any more rubbish in her life because I'm finally listening and I'm awake and present and ready to be me. I can truly have it all!

Thank you for allowing me to share part of my story with you. I don't share it for any type of sympathy. I share it because, as the name of this chapter suggests, I've done it the hard way and I'd really love to make it easier for you.

EXERCISE PATH TO SPIRITUALITY

Here are some exercises you can try to wake up to consciousness.

1- Practice Mindfulness

As I said earlier, this could be as simple as how you eat or how you happen to walk to work. If you haven't figured it out already, I'm a big fan of multitasking since time can seem so limited. There are some great books you can read on mindfulness. One of my favorites is Ruby Wax's book, *A Mindfulness Guide for the Frazzled*, which is a really easy read with great exercises.

You can get coloring books that are specifically designed for mindfulness and have incredibly intricate drawings. Spending time focusing on coloring tiny little patterns forces you to pay attention to that, rather than allowing your mind to be distracted by your surroundings. Again, if you want to multitask, I love to color sitting down with my seven-year-old while the other two are watching TV or sometimes even for 10 minutes during my lunch break or on the train to work. Again, be creative in how you incorporate mindfulness into your everyday life.

2- Listen

Sometimes we ask people to be quiet so that we can hear. Well, the same goes for your life. Take a bit of time out each day to avoid being distracted by cell phones, social media conversations, and give yourself some quiet time in order to truly hear. The only way you can hear yourself is to drown out the noise.

Meditation is not the easiest thing to do. Usually when we decide to take action, we expect to physically be doing something, but meditation is about being still. When you're first starting out with meditation, practice a chant that drowns out the surrounding noise. Place your thumb and middle finger together and become aware of the pressure that this creates. This drowns out the mental noise and helps you to focus, so that you can then "defocus" while meditating. Practicing breathing in and out over several counts and focusing on your breath also helps. Some people like to stare at a candle and their thoughts eventually subside so they can then hear themselves. You don't even need to be sitting still. You can meditate while walking, which just means walking without allowing other distractions. I often find myself meditating when I'm working out because the exercise becomes so automatic that I shut off the background noise and hear myself in the thoughts and inspirations that pop into my head from nowhere. Inspiration means "in spirit."

Guided meditations are a great way to get started until you increase your skill level. There are countless apps available that can help with this.

To help you get started, download a quick five-minute centering guided meditation exercise from the book resources section of www.lightchangescoaching.com. Just doing this five-minute exercise at the start of your day can be powerful and get you to start listening to yourself.

3- Trust

This ties into hearing yourself. Trust what you hear. Trust your gut instinct and try your best to follow it. Consider that when something becomes too hard and it seems barriers are being put in the way left, right, and center, maybe there's a reason for that. It could be that path isn't the right one to take. Look for signs all around that are guiding you to go in a particular direction and really try to engage with your gut, feeling and follow it. Again, meditation helps you to develop this skill over time.

4- Change Your Vocabulary

This exercise is really great for empowering you to recognize that you have a choice in everything. If you choose to do something, then that effectively means you are making a conscious choice to do it and therefore are aligning with your values and your true self rather than feeling that you have to. Start off small. It might be making yourself a cup of tea in the morning and thinking "I choose to drink my tea" and then other things that you do every day, like:

o   "I choose to go to work"

o   "I choose to exercise"

o   "I choose to eat healthily"

o   "I choose to spend two hours on social media tonight"

o   "I choose to eat that huge slice of chocolate cake, and to hell with the consequences"

o   "I choose to prepare that presentation for tomorrow's meeting," and so on.

You get the idea. It's about shifting your mindset from having to do something or feeling guilty about doing something, to actually making a choice to do it. That choice then gives you power.

Let's go back to the chocolate cake. Think of how much more enjoyment you're going to have by choosing to have the chocolate cake and choosing not to feel guilty about it and therefore how much more mindful you're going to be and how you're going to enjoy every single moment rather than worrying about what the consequences will be.

Think of a presentation you have to do for work. Well, you have a deadline, so it has to be done. You can sit there procrastinating and feeling resentful. Or you can make a conscious choice to choose to do it and in so doing, rather than wasting the time with anger and resentment about it, you'll probably get it done in much less time, and then have other time to actually enjoy things. It's a little bit like gratitude. As you start to incorporate choice more into your life, you'll step more into your own power and start choosing much bigger things and making much more impactful decisions that align with yourself.

It will lift your energy!

5- Learn More About Yourself

When it comes to trying to find your actual life purpose or identifying exactly what your beliefs are and overcoming blocks and fears, hiring the right coach can be really helpful.

#Insights

CHAPTER 3

BOUNDARIES:
DO YOU EVEN KNOW WHAT THEY ARE?

*"Your personal boundaries protect the inner core of your identity and
your right to choices."*
~ Gerard Manley Hopkins

According to the *Oxford Dictionary*, the word 'boundary' is defined as "a
line which marks the limit of an area, a dividing line." If we can see
boundaries on the cricket pitch and we can see them as the fences
between our houses, then why do we not see them in our own lives?

A personal boundary is a physical, emotional, or mental limit which is
established to protect oneself from being manipulated, used, or
violated by others. If you're anything like me, and I think women often
fall into this category more than men, we often do things to please
other people and put other people's needs before our own. "Where's
the harm in that?" I hear you say. "It's good to do things for other

people. It makes me feel good knowing that I've made people happy. I couldn't possibly be selfish enough to put myself first." However, there is actually a difference between putting yourself first and not putting yourself in the equation at all.

Have you ever felt taken for granted at home by your partner or children or maybe in the workplace by your colleagues who always dump on you? They may ask you to be the spokesperson of the group because they've defined you as the person who can organize everybody. You step into that role even though you may not actually truly be comfortable with it, because it's something you've always done. If you've let that go on for years, you can imagine the repercussions if you suddenly find your voice again and say, "Well, actually, I don't want to be the one organizing everybody. I'd like someone else to do it for a change." My former husband often used to blame those sudden outbursts on my hormones and time of the month and so I would quietly retreat and do what was expected of me.

To give you another personal example, when we went on holiday when our children were young I would spend hours packing, making sure we had all the medicines and clothes for all eventualities as one does with young kids. Then, every morning, I would pack up the beach bags. When we got back from swimming all day, I was the one hanging out all the swimsuits, putting the after-sun lotion on all the kids, getting myself ready for dinner and then being told off for being late. All the while my kids were having the best of times, not the slightest bit aware that their mother was stressed, and my husband was sitting on a bed enjoying a good book or playing some game on his phone. I, in the meantime, would be bubbling with frustration and anger at nobody helping me, but in actual fact, had I ever actually voiced the need for help? No! Was I seen as supermom and super wife? Yes, absolutely! Did it serve me well? No!

I go back to that tragic experience of abuse in my childhood and not having a voice. I was upset and hurt by other people's responses to my grandfather's abuse after I told them about it, but not once did I voice what my expectations were or how I expected them to stand up for me and how I deserved that.

This is something we so commonly do. We just automatically expect other people to understand us and behave in the way that we want them to. It's the classic "treat people how you expect to be treated," but believe it or not, people don't always respond in quite the same way. An article by Z. Hereford in "Essential Life Skills" lists some signs of unhealthy boundaries, which I think you'll find really useful:

a) going against personal values or rights in order to please others

b) giving as much as you can for the sake of giving

c) taking as much as you can for the sake of taking

d) letting others define you

e) expecting others to fill your needs automatically

f) feeling bad or guilty when you say no

g) not speaking up when you're treated poorly

h) falling apart so someone can take care of you

i) falling in love with someone you barely know or who reaches out to you

j) accepting advances or any kind of touching that you don't want

k) touching a person without asking

I don't know about you, but a few years ago I could certainly relate to more than three quarters of those signs of unhealthy boundaries. I allowed other people to define me. We start to derive our sense of self-worth from those people. Have you ever felt guilty when somebody gives you a hugely expensive gift and yet you yourself would have been delighted to have given them the same gift? If that's the case, then think where your sense of self-worth must be when you feel you're undeserving of that present. Have you ever gone out with your friends even though you didn't really want to, but you worried about what they might think of you or didn't want to let them down?

Have you ever ordered a dessert that you didn't really want or gone out drinking to make the people around you feel more comfortable, rather than truly pleasing yourself? Have you ever become the victim at work where you're plied with more and more work and yet no one seems to recognize the stress you're under? Have you found yourself cutting down to a four-day week only to actually have five days' worth of work to do in that time? Where was your voice on any of those occasions? Why were you worried about what other people think? And if you really go a little bit deeper, how worth it are those people if they don't allow you to be you?

Now, I understand that it will take quite a lot of delving and self-discovery to clearly tell yourself "I deserve better" and feel brave about it. But the more you start to step into your true self and align yourself with your values, the more that statement will align with your behavior.

EXERCISE PATH TO ESTABLISHING HEALTHY BOUNDARIES

1- Drawing The Boundary Lines

This first exercise will help you to identify where your boundaries lie. I'm a huge fan of lists. So here's a list for you. I invite you to think about what you are and are not prepared to accept in other people's behavior towards you. It sounds so obvious, but until you start writing it down, you may not really clearly see what you're tolerating and accepting in your life that you're not actually happy about. I'll walk you through the full exercise and there's a great worksheet you can download from www.lightchangescoaching.com to help you work your way through it.

Draw three columns. The first column is for you to list everything you are prepared to accept in your life. This might be things like hugs, cups of tea made for you, compliments, words of encouragement, constructive criticism, or even diamonds!

Leave the next column blank and move straight on to the third column which is about everything you are presently unwilling to accept. That might be things like insults, poor communication, lack of appreciation, inappropriate touching, lack of recognition, etc.

The middle column, not surprisingly, is a gray area. These are the aspects you might be willing to meet in the middle on, or tolerate. So you might find these are a little bit harder to write concisely because you might want to add scenarios to them. For example, "I'm prepared to tolerate my partner coming home really late from work as long as he makes sure that he doesn't work over the weekends and we get to spend quality time together." Or it might be something like "I'm prepared to work through my lunch break as long as I get to leave work early."

In working through these three lists, you may want to go back and question them as you reflect on them and see if certain items really do belong in a particular category or if they need to be shifted into another column.

Once your lists are complete, grade the things in your list based on how often they happen in your life. So on a scale of 1 to 10, where 10 is the most often and 1 is the least often, work your way through the list. It's a good idea to start with the list of things you are absolutely not prepared to tolerate. Needless to say, if you start finding you are grading most of the things on that list between scores of 7 and 10, then you're quite clearly not honoring your boundaries. This is an incredibly powerful exercise which puts down on paper what's going on in your life and starts to give you a sense of awareness about your circumstances. If in doing this exercise you recognize that you already have healthy boundaries, then good for you. That's absolutely wonderful and I fully congratulate you! I wish it hadn't taken me 40-plus years to get to that stage.

Drawing The Boundary Lines

What Am I Prepared To Accept?	G R A D E	What Would A Win-Win Middle Ground Look Like For Me?	G R A D E	What Am I Unwilling To Accept?	G R A D E

The next stage after identifying where your boundaries lie is to communicate them.

2- Communication

This can seem like an incredibly scary task, but until you start honoring yourself, no one is going to do it for you. I always remember getting myself really worked up before I had to have a conversation with my husband about something I wasn't happy about. I was conscious of not wanting to seem like a nag and wanting my needs to be heard and met, which meant really trying to get him to listen beneath the surface of what I was actually saying.

When I told him I really didn't want him going straight to the pub after work because that was about six o'clock and it was time to put the children to bed, I wasn't saying I wanted to spoil his fun and his relaxation time. In actual fact, I was communicating my need to have help with our children, who were still babies. Of course, it never really came out that way. It came out as me screaming, "Why do you always go to the pub?! I'm the one left putting the kids to bed and I'm the one who can't go to the gym and exercise because you always choose that time and I'm the one who ends up cooking dinner and I'm exhausted and I've had a long day at work too!" Woe was me as I fully engaged in playing the role of the victim. How could I possibly expect a change in my husband's behavior if I made it so clear I was willing to tolerate that behavior and also didn't truly express my underlying needs, which would have appealed to his much more loving and compassionate side?

Another example of communication pertains to how we bring up our children. So often we make threats about what will happen if they don't behave in a certain way, but then there's no follow-through. How are children supposed to learn where our boundaries lie if we don't define them clearly enough? My 12-year-old knows I mean business when he doesn't come downstairs to have dinner because he's playing on his gaming PC. If I've called him for the third time, that computer gets put away for a week! He's learned to understand where my boundaries lie and how he can't take advantage of my good nature. That doesn't mean that I don't love him and he doesn't love me. Over time we've built up not only a huge amount of affection for each other, but also an effective, strong relationship rich in communication. He in turn has set his own boundaries with me in that I know not to embarrass him in front of his friends, for example, and I don't start singing when I go to wake him up in the morning as it just puts him in a bad mood.

There are some great books that you might find helpful when it comes to communicating where your boundaries lie with people. One is called *The Five Love Languages* by Gary Chapman. He's written several other books to do with five languages in the workplace, five languages of communication, five languages with children, with teenagers, with men, with women, and so on. But the principles are that in the same way we may speak either French, English, Arabic, Russian, we also speak love in different ways. He outlines the five principle ways of expressing love as:

- o Words of affirmation – for example, someone saying they love you.

- o Receiving gifts from someone – someone expresses their love by giving you presents, and you feel loved by receiving those.

- o Acts of service – I know in my case my husband felt he was showing his love by how well he was looking after the house, mowing the lawn, and doing the chores.

- o Quality time – this involves being able to spend quality time with somebody and feeling truly loved because of it.

- o Physical touch – for example, somebody feels loved when they're hugging or kissing or holding hands.

Understanding your personal primary love language can be really helpful in learning to communicate with other people around you. Though you may feel completely taken for granted at work, your boss may think she is showing her appreciation and admiration by sending you her most high-profile clients because she knows that you can handle them. If you haven't told your boss that you need to hear that kind of praise and would like to receive bonuses, then you're both speaking different languages and no boundaries have been defined because you are accepting the situation as it stands.

Another book packed with useful tips is *Non-Violent Communication* by Marshall Rosenberg. It teaches you how to effectively communicate your needs. Once you identify those needs, then you're also identifying the boundaries of what you are and are not prepared to accept.

3- Walking The Talk

Having identified where your boundaries actually lie and what you are and are not prepared to tolerate, the next step is to truly trust and believe in who you are. This goes back to the previous chapter about consciousness and knowing your values and living a life that aligns with them. It's about stepping into your own power and making decisions about yourself, *for* yourself. For example, you may have a preference for more of a vegetarian diet while the rest of your family eats anything. In cooking meat for them, you may then also go along with eating food that doesn't necessarily make you feel great. By doing that, you're not aligning with your value of healthy eating as you perceive it. In this example, you may not have set the boundary and are therefore allowing others to define you and doing things to please everybody else rather than yourself.

Once you recognize that, you may find a middle ground of preparing a vegetarian meal perhaps half of the week, and making it clear exactly why you're doing that, in which case you hope that other people will honor your need as you have honored theirs. If they don't, that's another conversation to be had, which we'll talk about later in this book.

Unless you start to honor your own needs, how is anyone else expected to do that for you? What starts to happen is that we rely on external rewards to make us feel happy. When there's an imbalance of not truly being ourselves, we can start to become needy by relying on the praise of others to feel good about ourselves, for example, or wanting to be the rescuer who solves everybody's problems and feels better about it. But that constant giving will drain you in the end because you get nothing back in return.

In core-energy™ coaching, we talk about a few particular levels of energy that relate to these circumstances. Level 4 is called service energy, where we want to give all the time. But like I said, if all you do is give, give, give, in the end you will be drained and there'll be nothing left in the tank. As we move up to Level 5 it becomes more of a win-win situation. Think of an example such as "I make dinner for you one night and you make dinner for me. We'll both benefit, which potentially is a much healthier response."

It gets even better if we move up to Level 6, which becomes an everybody-wins situation. So if we're sticking with eating, we might decide that we'll cook together in which case we have the benefit of enjoying quality time together, input into what the meal is going to be, both being engaged in the task, and both enjoying the meal because we've taken the time to prepare it for each other. In core-energy coaching™, we aim to coach you from Level 1, which is the victim stage, right up to Level 7, which allows you to feel joyful, purposeful, and more!

When we possess healthy personal boundaries, then we have more stability and control over our own lives. We have better, more fulfilling relationships, both intimate, social, and in the workplace. We are better able to communicate with each other. We are more in touch with reality. We have improved self-confidence, self-esteem, and self-perception. We have more energy, both emotional and physical.

For years I had so much difficulty saying 'no' to anything and would work myself into the ground because I took on so much and felt guilty about not pleasing my partner, my children, my siblings, my father, and my employees. I put all of them before myself. It was only after going to a workshop with some really useful physical exercises that the penny finally dropped and I learned how to say 'no' and in fact how *good* it felt to say no. It was a tantra workshop, so there was touching involved, albeit fully clothed, and people were in turn allowed to touch us.

As the blindfolded person, or person with their eyes closed, as was the case with me, you had the power to say, "Number one, you may touch me," and that person might stroke your hair, face, or arm. You were allowed to say if you wanted more of it; less; if you wanted them to stop; or if it was unacceptable that they touched you somewhere you weren't comfortable. You could then invite a second person to do the same either simultaneously or individually. The process could be repeated with a third person. It was unbelievable how much control I suddenly felt by the fact that I could say, "No! This is not okay! I don't want it!"

It was a workshop full of these types of exercises where I made a conscious choice about what I did and didn't want to do. Nothing happened to me. I wasn't suddenly cast aside or ridiculed for stating my boundaries. It's something that seems so simple and yet in reality is so hard for most of us.

Simply put: *How can we expect people to respect us if we don't respect ourselves?*

Boundaries allow us to separate who we are and what we think we need and want, from the thoughts, feelings, and opinions of others. They help us be our true selves and enable us to allow the same in others.

Other useful ideas for you to put into action:

1- I realize a lot in this chapter may seem easier said than done, but just start by doing the first exercise and take baby steps. It might help to get a friend to help you out in terms of accountability. Tell them how you're going to define a boundary in a particular aspect, which might mean a conversation with your boss, partner, or child. Have that friend hold you accountable to make sure the conversation actually happens.

2- Try journaling – making bold statements about who you are and how you expect and deserve to be treated. Just writing these down and reading them ultimately allows you to give off the energy of what you've written and so you'll naturally start to emanate that energy even if you haven't verbalized it.

3- Go back to the mirror exercise we talked about in the last chapter and add in statements such as "I respect myself," "I won't be taken for granted," "It's not okay to be treated a certain way," etc.

4- You could also do the Four Phrases exercise in this respect. Think about a boundary that's being overstepped that's making you unhappy. It might be something like your boss expecting you to work late but not paying you overtime. In recognizing that this is overstepping your boundaries, say, *"I'm sorry,"* meaning you are sorry for not recognizing it before. *"Please forgive me"* means you want to forgive yourself for the fact that you haven't honored your boundaries. *"Thank you"* is for allowing yourself the space to recognize this and have this realization and the fact that things are about to change. And *"I love you"* means that you love, respect, and honor yourself.

Lastly, get comfortable with saying *it's not okay* and use the words as soon as your boundaries are overstepped.

Summary for #Women Who Want More

I invite you to consider the following in helping you to work on your boundaries:

- list your boundaries so that you can identify exactly what you are and aren't prepared to tolerate in your life

- communicate them directly to those around you

- keep working on yourself to know who you are, what your values are, and walk the talk.

- use all this to write your new rule book. We all have an unconscious rule book for how we live our lives, but it is unlikely that we have ever really taken the time to write it down. Creating your rule book based on what you are learning, who you are becoming, and how you want to live your life can help propel you in that direction. It is about making conscious decisions and choices.

Now that we've laid the foundations of working out who you are and loving it, let's discuss some specifics of how to create a fulfilled and balanced life.

#Insights

CHAPTER 4

BE A LEADER
AND WEAR A SKIRT

"A woman with a voice is by definition a strong woman. But the search to find that voice can be remarkably difficult."
~ Melinda Gates

What does it mean to be a leader? Are you one? Do you want to be one? Do you compromise your femininity in order to be one? Have you noticed how most of us tend to define ourselves by what we do rather than who we are? When we first meet somebody, "So what do you do for a living?" is often one of the first questions we ask. We may not even be interested in the answer; it's just a way of starting conversation. Have you noticed how the reply usually starts with the phrase "I am"? Here's a question for you: Are you really? Are you really a lawyer? Are you really a teacher? Are you really a banker or a business owner or an entrepreneur or a beautician or a doctor? Is there more to you or is that truly all that defines you? I hope that in asking that question you recognize what I'm getting at. You may be one of those things or something else but that's what you do, not who you are.

My next question is: What do you do? You may be a homemaker, but what exactly do you *do*? Your response may be that you look after the home, making sure that it's a peaceful, welcoming, safe environment for yourself and/or your family; you may be a personal trainer and help people achieve their physical fitness goals. Hopefully by now you're starting to get my gist in that, while your response to my second question may tell me a little bit more about you, it still doesn't really tell me who you are. It can be a fun way to respond to "What do you do?" by using a more descriptive form rather than labeling yourself, so I'd invite you to give it a try next time you're asked.

When people ask me what it is I do, I respond: I help people get 'unstuck' and empower them to be their true selves.

Now consider your life purpose. Your purpose in life may not be your profession or whatever you happen to do for a living. Another way to look at life purpose is to consider that it is about doing everything in your life purposefully. It's a great shame if you spend at least eight hours a day doing something that doesn't give you any fulfillment, but the reality is that is so often the case. However, the good news is it doesn't have to be!

Have you noticed how you can strive towards one thing in the true belief that when you have it, it will make you be happy? "I'll be happy when I get that job." You put your energy into that; may or may not, as is often the case, take the time to celebrate; then move onto the next thing. "Okay, I got the job, but I'm not as happy as I thought I'd be. I know—I'll be happy when I have a partner." So you pursue the perfect partner, are happy for a while, but then once again, the same thing happens. You chase the perfect body, then money, then another job, then a child, then a lifetime ambition, then a house, and so it goes on. Constantly seeking happiness. Constantly seeking purpose to find that feeling of fulfillment. How wonderful would it be if the purpose and fulfillment was within us and we could tap into ourselves to feel it, rather than pursuing it through externals, be that people, places, or things?

I would urge you to consider being a leader in whatever it is you do. A leader doesn't necessarily mean being a boss, or needing to be bossy. It means self-mastery. It means being able to perform any tasks to the best of your ability with enthusiasm, high energy, and high productivity. It means inspiring others. A leader is solution-focused in solving problems. Leaders are dynamic, able to communicate effectively, have a high degree of emotional intelligence, and are able to manage and balance multiple tasks. They can be and do all this while remaining healthy and true to themselves and feeling purposeful.

"Wow!" I hear you say. "That doesn't sound very simple or easy to achieve!"

Nobody said anything about this process would be easy, but the rewards when you manage it are priceless. It took me a long time to understand that I could be a leader without needing to own a business. I was a periodontist for 15 years, and built up two clinics, one of which I sold, and the other I set up when my second child was just two months old. That clinic grew from strength to strength and got busier and busier, to the point where it started to control me rather than the other way around.

To add to that, I have always been somebody who is very forward-thinking and innovative, and so I started to incorporate a new type of technology that meant we were able to treat patients in an incredibly minimally invasive way. This propelled my career in another direction where I found myself working with companies in the US on product development and marketing; helping universities develop research protocols; teaching and training colleagues all around the world; running courses; and being invited as a keynote speaker on the global stage several times a year. In a field that is largely dominated by men, I had no issue with being the only woman on the program and felt no pressure to be like them—I was quite happy wearing a skirt. I had three children, a home life, friends, financial responsibilities, and a husband to all satisfy at the same time. To say there was an imbalance in all of this would be an understatement. But so unfulfilled was I in some of the other aspects of my life that I sought complete fulfillment from just one source, which was work.

There was no time for fun and relaxation—I was just on a treadmill, allowing my career to control me, and to some extent I became a victim of my own success. While the clinic was doing incredibly well, always busy with new patients, and I had a loyal staff, a great reputation, and ever-increasing revenue where we doubled the turnover each year for the last two years, I was still there for several hours after everybody else had gone home. That wasn't life. My children needed me. *I* needed me, but I was nowhere to be found.

I couldn't bring myself to let go of that business because that was what I felt defined me. It was only following a session with my coach that I finally realized I could be a leader without needing to be the boss. I was still a leader in my field, but in letting go of what was making me unhappy, and in identifying what was truly important to me, I made space for fulfillment. Space to find me again. Space to be free.

I should add here that my income didn't go down when I sold my clinic. In fact, it went up because not only was I doing what I loved—helping and teaching people—but I had so much more energy and balance in my life.

Why is being a leader so important?

As we've already discussed, a leader encompasses someone who is:

- o   authentic

- o   able to practice self-mastery

- o   solution-focused

- o emotionally intelligent

- o able to engage in high-energy relationships

- o inspirational

- o motivational

- o enthusiastic

- o highly productive

- o good in communication

- o dynamic

- o outward-thinking

- o observant

- o responsive

- o able to manage and balance multiple tasks

Its significance comes back to energy levels. In the last chapter I noted that when we are in Level 1 energy of being in victim mode where we allow everything to control us, then we can become very insular. This means everything is happening *to* us rather than *for* us, and we have no control. Or we think we don't. The number of clients I have come across in these types of situations is vast. When I ask them about their work life, they feel completely overwhelmed. This might be due to the workload itself or lack of time to be able to do it; it might mean a lack of understanding from their line managers, superiors, or bosses when it comes to the pressure that they are putting on their employees or a missing awareness of their employees' circumstances and needs. It's certainly not a win-win situation. It is a draining situation, one that lacks fulfillment and creates stress.

When I ask patients about their stress levels before treatment, it's very rare to find a retiree who doesn't say his or her stress levels have gone down considerably since leaving the rat race. In the UK alone, 15.4 million workdays were lost in 2017-2018 due to stress, depression, and anxiety, with an average of each person suffering stress taking 25.8 days off, according to the Health and Safety Executive 2017-18 data.

How great would it be to be working, loving what you do, feeling able to cope with it, even looking forward to it every day, and feeling no stress whatsoever? Priceless or what?!

The secret is mindset.

How can you incorporate the aspects of leadership into whatever it is you do?

Let me share the story of one of my clients who was a banker before she had children. She quit working in order to devote her time to her children as her husband also had a high-end job and she felt that at least one parent needed to be home, and it made more sense for her to give up her job as she didn't earn as much. This is not uncommon among middle-class professionals. My client felt inferior because she wasn't bringing money into the household. Even her children saw her as inferior to some extent, or so she thought. When her kids grew up and left home for college, she was suddenly left with very little identity at all. Who was she? What skills did she have? What was she going to do with the rest of her life? Sure, they had money, but that wasn't going to fulfill her need for a purpose. She suddenly found herself with plenty of time, something she had craved so desperately just a short while before, but nothing to fill it with.

This is a classic example of imbalance where someone has health, time, money, friends, a loving husband and family, but no feeling of life purpose, which leads to a lack of identity and self-mastery. How could I help her be a leader in her life? To start, she needed to reframe things in her mind and not feel inferior for having been a homemaker. She needed to take control of her life again and instead of thinking her husband and children made her feel inferior and that her role was less important, she needed to understand that she had chosen to feel that way. What we choose to think is based on our experiences and perceptions and how we view the world, and quite clearly in her case there was an element of not truly believing in the importance of the role that she was playing in the home. She therefore assumed that others didn't believe in it either. Reframing her self-belief opened up her mind and her ability to see opportunities more clearly. It allowed her to redefine her boundaries, engage with her intuition, identify her unique skills, believe in herself, and start showing up more energetically. By radiating high levels of energy she was able to shift from victim to master. She became a leader of her family and herself and went on to establish a successful business using the skills acquired over a lifetime.

One of the foundational principles introduced to me during my core-energy™ coach training was 'energy attracts like energy.' I like to think of it as sitting in the middle of a lake surrounded by mountains. If I sing out loud, then that noise will echo off the mountains and reflect back to me. This is a great principle to apply within the workplace. If we show up as our true, beautiful, inspiring, and energetic selves, then that will reflect back to us from the people and environment around us. If we show up feeling put-upon, thinking we are being picked on or passed up for promotion, it's probably because that is the energy we are giving off—one of un-deservedness.

Returning to my own example of my work life when I ran my clinic—all of my staff would go above and beyond for me, each other, and our patients and referring practitioners. It wasn't all about the money that they were being paid. They would stay late after work, come in on their days off, work through their lunch breaks, and on most days had a smile on their faces. I led by example both in terms of my commitment and also the unstoppable smile on my own face. I inspired my team and they inspired me. I communicated my needs to them and they in turn allowed me to meet their needs, both through direct communication and my intuitiveness. This is all indicative of a high-energy working environment.

What happened when I sold my business to a corporation was both interesting and saddening. They came in without listening to the needs of staff, without understanding what it was that made our clinic and service unique, what it was that worked well and what didn't work so well, all of which we could have told them as we already knew. Within the first year the corporation redecorated the practice, set up a new website that was difficult and confusing to navigate, ignored any feedback, gave everybody a pay raise, and lost most of the long-term staff. Those that stayed clocked in and clocked out at the exact hours they were paid for.

This is an example of a low-energy working environment where the team was no longer engaged, people no longer felt listened to or appreciated, their jobs were not understood nor valued, and the duties they were given were not tailored to their specific skill-set. Where was the leadership?

If we apply the principle of "energy attracts like energy" then the new business owners had low energy levels and this was reflected back to them. It's not at all an uncommon situation with mergers and takeovers.

How does this relate to you if you don't own a business? Even if you're not the boss, if you engage in the leadership that we've been talking about, and you start to give off higher levels of energy, those around you will be affected and hopefully lift their energy levels as a result of your influence. At the very least you may recognize your own worth. If you determine that the people you work with don't deserve you, you may choose to move on elsewhere. If you shift who you are inside, and value your worth, then you will shift the situation and people around you.

EXERCISE PATH TO BECOMING A LEADER

Robin Sharma writes about leadership beautifully in his book *The Leader Who Had No Title*. This encompasses exactly what we've been talking about, which is transcending the ego and showing up as your true, authentic self. Whatever your role happens to be, if you can identify your purpose within that role, then fulfillment will follow.

1- Powerful Questions

Let me ask you the following questions. Try to jot down the first answers that come into your head as those are frequently the most heartfelt ones, before you have time to override them with logic and "ifs" and "buts."

- What feeling do you repeatedly have on a daily basis when you start your day?

- Where do you have this feeling in your body?

- How do you feel in the middle of the day?

- How do you feel at the end of the day?

- What opportunities for learning present themselves during the day?

- What's the first phrase you say to yourself as you start your workday?

- What's the last phrase you say to yourself as you end your workday?

- How much control do you feel you have during your workday?

- Are you working to live or living to work?

- When you feel you've had a great day, what are the top three things that needed to happen for you to define it as successful?

This exercise is a really useful way of reflecting back to yourself what is going on in your mind and body. If you start your day feeling anxiety, that's an energy you're giving off. If you end your day feeling exhausted and deflated, then there are clues in that as to what happened during the day and why. If you're telling yourself that today is going to be stressful, then it's no surprise that you're giving off the energy and expectation of being stressed, in which case you usually will be.

On the other hand, if you're telling yourself it's going to be a great, hassle-free, exciting high-energy day, the chances are it will be. If you don't feel in control of your day at work, then that's a clue that you haven't effectively defined your boundaries and there may be a communication issue. If you haven't noticed any opportunities for growth, then again, this is telling you that you are operating from a lower energy level because as we move up the energy scale we are open to all opportunities for growth no matter the job. If you're working to live or living to work, both are indicative of an imbalance.

That final question, "When you feel you've had a great day, what are the top three things that needed to happen for you to define it as successful?", will help you to identify three of your most important needs in your workday. Keep in mind that when I'm talking about workday I mean typical day-to-day duties. These apply even if you don't have a job that generates income at this point in time. It may be useful to go back to these questions in a few months' time after you've done the work on yourself and see how the answers differ.

2- Write Your Own Ad

Write your own job advertisement. This helps to set your focus and intention. You don't need to say what it is for, such as a doctor or hairdresser. Write the ad based on the skills needed and the aspects of your personality that would get you the job.

1- List the skills you possess and what you want people to see in you.

2- Suggest a salary of whatever you feel you are worth. Don't undervalue yourself.

3- List the benefits the person applying would expect to get if hired.

4- Write down the opportunities that are available. Make sure you're thinking about what it is you would want.

5- Explain how to apply for the job.

Once you're finished, print out the ad and place it somewhere highly visible. Below I have given you an example of a job ad I wrote for myself.

HELP WANTED

Someone who has the ability to see the best in others, engage in their creativity, inspire and be inspired, work with the team, communicate effectively, be innovative, dynamic, well-organized, who has high-level authenticity, values excellence, listens, has the ability to prioritize, is solution-focused, works towards a common goal, respects all those around them and themselves, responds versus reacts, thinks outside the box, values health and self-care, is ethical, is able to bring a wealth of life experience, and is unafraid to show up every day expressing all of these qualities.

Salary: Why be limited by a number! Incredibly high because I'm worth it.

Benefits: The successful candidate will have so much fulfillment. They will wake up in the morning feeling as energetic as when they leave at the end of the day and always feel in full and complete control of every situation they may encounter. Their health and well-being will be looked after and their abilities will be fully nurtured. They will never feel alone.

Opportunity: For continued growth advancement and self-mastery.

How to apply: Look within yourself!

Just writing the ad down, regardless of what it looks like on paper, shifts your energy in order to think about who you truly are and how you want to appear during the day.

So often we undervalue ourselves not only emotionally but monetarily. I myself did this for years. I told you about the innovative treatment that I was doing in my clinic and how I became the first specialist carrying out such treatments in the UK and then became a global leader in that particular field. And yet I charged very little in comparison to my colleagues who were not performing the same procedure. Even in my speaking engagements, I would accept very low fees in comparison to most of my colleagues. Part of this admittedly was because I had a different mission and a different purpose—not so much the need to earn more money, but the increasing opportunity to influence key people and open their minds up to possibilities. I was on a mission to open the eyes of my profession and transform it.

I also told you how I was frequently the only woman on stage. Women frequently experience something called "imposter syndrome." Listening to people talking about my course or the lecture I had just given, describing it as one of the best they had ever attended, I would wonder who on earth they were talking about. There was a disconnect between who I was inside and how I was valuing myself compared to how I was showing up as a confident, self-assured teacher and speaker. The fact that I hadn't defined my boundaries meant that I found myself with no voice to shout out, "But of course I deserve to be paid highly! You just need to listen to the feedback from the attendees to know that!" Instead, I hoped that someone else would say it for me. But the energy I was emanating was one of "I don't deserve anything more." I was telling the universe being undervalued was okay.

Some years ago, while being coached myself, we role-played the ability to ask for more money for a speaking engagement. I also had to put strategies in place to get my team on board within the clinic to make sure that they all believed in the high value of what we were offering so that when we then asked for fees, patients were happy to pay them because we ourselves were giving off the energy of truly believing in the value of what we had to offer. Yes, you have to look people in the eye; yes, you have to engage with them, and all the other things a marketing company may teach you when it comes to asking for payment, but without true self-belief, it is worthless. This is really the key. You have to believe in what you're offering. You have to believe in yourself. You have to give off that energy of belief and the only way to do it is to have it deep within yourself.

3- 7 Days To Being A Leader

The final exercise will help you identify your purpose and will help you to apply that purpose to your workday with passion and leadership. Definitely download the worksheet for this as it is something you will want to record over the course of a week. I call this exercise *7 Days to Being a Leader*, and you can download it by visiting www.lightchangescoaching.com.

Draw three columns. In the first column, list what it means to you to be a leader based on your beliefs and include some of the takeaways you've gathered from this chapter. We've talked about the need to be authentic, practice self-mastery, be solution-focused, have emotional intelligence, have high energy, be inspirational, etc. Take a little bit of time to list the characteristics of what being a leader means to you.

In the next column, on a scale from 1 to 10, 10 being the most often and 1 the least, rate how often a particular characteristic shows up in your day.

In the final column, list how you might be able to demonstrate those skills within your day. Do this for a one-week period. Use the worksheets you printed off so you can put your score from 1 to 10 in each day of the week.

Let's look at another client of mine who was a creative director with her own business. One of the aspects of leadership that appealed to her was being able to engage and influence others. For one week while working on a project, each day she rated how effectively and often she was demonstrating that skill. She also listed examples of how she might use that skill. In her case she listed things such as the ability to inspire and get her team to be enthusiastic about her creative suggestions, the ability to get her team to follow through the work she had outlined, and the ability to convert leads into clients. This is a sample of how she recorded it:

Desired Leadership Skill	How Often Does It Show Up? (scale 1-10)	How Does It Show Up?
Engage and influence others	Monday: 3 Tuesday: 5 Wednesday: 4	Convert leads into real clients Get team on board with creative ideas

After one week, she realized that she was rating this desired leadership skill of engaging and influencing others as very low and this in turn helped her to recognize that it was leading to a great deal of dissatisfaction within her work role. We were then able to explore further as to what blocks might be stopping her from showing up with the skill that she so desired.

When you do the initial exercise to gain awareness, ask yourself what is stopping you from demonstrating those skills and how you can change it. My client described "productivity" as achieving all the tasks necessary, meeting deadlines, and answering new leads. All these characteristics were rated very highly in her chart. She was clearly demonstrating leadership in being highly productive, but because there was an imbalance within her leadership, she was still feeling unfulfilled and stressed. Once we identified the pieces that were missing within her definition of leadership, that helped her to engage in those areas more energetically, so she shifted into higher levels of fulfillment, self-worth, and self-value.

7 Days To Being A Leader

Desired Leadership Skill	How Often Does It Show Up? (scale 1-10)	How Does It Show Up?
	Monday: Tuesday: Wednesday: Thursday: Friday: Saturday: Sunday:	
	Monday: Tuesday: Wednesday: Thursday: Friday: Saturday: Sunday:	
	Monday: Tuesday: Wednesday: Thursday: Friday: Saturday: Sunday:	
	Monday: Tuesday: Wednesday: Thursday: Friday: Saturday: Sunday:	

Summary for #Women Who Want More

I invite you to consider the following in trying to develop your leadership and master your skills:

- Explore how you want to present yourself to the world every day and make sure that you do

- Create an ad about the role you want to play in life, and keep it visible to remind you of how deserving you are

- Consider how you might master leadership in all aspects of your life, not just work

- Get people around you on board, including your work colleagues, your clients, and all your friends and family. Shout about how great you are!

- Take time to do the reflective work so that you can identify the key issues that influence your leadership

- Surround yourself with people who believe in you

- Consider finding a mentor who you can learn from

- Consider hiring a coach to help you and/or your team

#Insights

CHAPTER 5

PARENTAL BLISS:
I HAVE ONE, I AM ONE, I WANT TO BE ONE

*"Parents can only give good advice or put them on the right paths, but
the final forming of a person's character lies in their own hands."*
~ Anne Frank

Even in adulthood, do you find yourself wanting to seek approval from
your parents? Do you sometimes feel as if they're still treating you like
the child that you were rather than the adult you are now? Do you get
frustrated with them? Have you found that the roles have reversed and
now you need to look after them?

Are you a parent? How challenging is it to meet the needs of your child
or children while ensuring that your own needs are met? How much
fulfillment is being a parent giving you? Are you living your life through
your child's? How many sacrifices are you making in your life?

Are children even on the agenda? How high on the priority list are they? Are they even possible? What do you think having children will give you?

Having Parents

I recall a friend of mine saying that at some stage in adulthood you have to stop blaming your parents for everything and take responsibility for yourself. The reality is our parents all have to take a great deal of responsibility for how we grow up. It's usually their influences, belief systems, ideas, and rules that are passed down to us. As children we adopt the same beliefs until we become more conscious and start to see the world through our own eyes based on our own personal experiences. As we awaken and recognize that we have a choice in our beliefs, we may then choose to adopt some of those same beliefs from our childhood, and at the same time we may choose to shed some of them. It's all part of the growing-up process. The waking-up process. However, if nobody told our parents, how are they supposed to know how we have changed?

It's interesting to watch the dynamic as we grow up from being children who had to obey the rules, to becoming adults, then have the role reversed when we find ourselves parenting our parents. In so doing we give up our control because we go back to being that young child who is ever obedient and who forgets to be the grown-up. Or we try to be the grown-ups and it's not something our parents are used to, so we meet resistance from them. Why do we find that surprising? Our parents have always told us what to do and therefore they don't know any different. This becomes another source of stress where we feel that we are not heard or understood, that we're always trying to please, are not appreciated, or are being put upon. The difference, of course, is that as adults, we have other responsibilities which may include our working life, our friends, families, and other commitments, so time stress becomes a huge factor.

I personally have a wonderful relationship with my father, now in his seventies. Fortunately he's in good health and when he flies into the country to visit, I choose to drop other commitments to spend time with him. Having said that, at some point during the visit I'll feel some sense of exasperation that I am not being fully understood or heard. I still gauge what I say and tell him so that it works to my advantage in order to seek approval. I suppose I still want to remain on the pedestal that he put me on in childhood. I also get frustrated that while I may have prioritized my time to spend with him, he doesn't necessarily place the same priority on my free time and ends up letting me down. When this happens I feel frustrated and disrespected, but actually, he's just being himself and I just have to be me.

The key to having peace and harmony is to accept people as they are. We also have to try to understand where their behavior might be coming from, which in the case of my father is one of extreme love even though he doesn't share the same priorities as I do. Once I was able to resolve that in my head then I stopped getting so annoyed whenever his schedule changed. I didn't have to change who I was or how I behaved; it's just that my response was no longer an emotional one. This is very much about how, despite not being able to change the people or the situation, you can change the way you react, and with that comes freedom.

Let's talk a little bit more about belief systems. This is a good opportunity to introduce to you another one of iPEC's foundation principles:

"We are each a product of our own belief system."

Were you one of those children who was inspired to believe you could do anything and be anything? Were you encouraged to aim high? Were you made to feel special? If you were, the chances are you've then gone through life with a very similar attitude and have been able to integrate those beliefs into the person you've evolved into. For me, my mother led me to believe that I should always aim high and as an adult I've adopted the attitude of never doing anything by halves, so if I'm going to do something, I make sure I give it my all.

Conversely, if you've been told that you'll never be successful, that people like you never get such chances, or that you're not intelligent enough, then it will be much harder to overcome those beliefs and rebuild your self-esteem. One of my clients grew up with two older sisters and while they got all the attention, she adopted very strong beliefs that she would never make anything of her life because her sisters were the clever ones. She wasn't as pretty or as talented or anywhere near as special as them. She grew up with anxiety, a lack of self-belief, and anger issues, all to hide the deep insecurity within her. Years of counseling and therapy were unable to help with the anger, but just a few months of core-energy™ coaching saw her shift into somebody much calmer and happier. She became a leader and revealed her inner self to the outside world, which was someone full of kindness, love, and compassion who had been afraid to show up until then.

It's incredibly sad to think that our parents have this kind of influence on us. Righting those effects often requires a great deal of reconstruction in defining who we are.

EXERCISE PATH TO OVERCOMING PARENTAL INFLUENCES

Core-Belief Exercise

Like the other exercises in this book, feel free to download the worksheet from www.lightchangescoaching.com.

Divide your childhood into your first decade up to 10 years and your second decade up to age 20. Think about the beliefs that you had when you were a child. List them under the appropriate age column. Who gave you those beliefs?

Once you've put those beliefs down on paper and identified who was responsible for teaching them to you, decide how true those beliefs are for you today. To give you another example here, I grew up with the belief that I was always slightly on the pudgy side. My mother would put me on diets and relatives would frequently comment on my weight. Now, when I look back at that time, I have chosen not to carry that belief forward into my present-day life. Not only do I completely recognize that it wasn't true, but it also doesn't serve me in any way whatsoever. And so, in reflecting on the belief that played a role in my life from childhood, seeing how it may or may not have served me, thinking about how it might serve me now, and making a conscious choice as to whether or not I still choose to have that belief, I am giving myself back the control. I am giving myself the power.

Once you've written out your beliefs and decided whether you want to keep them or not, it's a good idea to actively write down your new beliefs. Take a past situation, for example. Maybe your dad always told you you were lazy when you were growing up. This may have been the case back then, but you may be incredibly hardworking now. A lot of the continued frustration with your dad may stem from the fact he inherently believes you're still lazy even though you're not. Understanding this can help you to feel less disturbed by such comments today. Then, by overwriting a past belief with another belief, which in this example is that you are incredibly hardworking, acknowledge that you may never be able to change your parents' opinion of you, but you in yourself will feel better because *you* know *your* truth.

It's not your role to change how other people think. It is much more powerful to change how *you* think. As you change the thoughts and beliefs around you, this will change how you feel about them and in turn it will shift your energy to bring about a different reality.

Decade Up To Age:

Core belief	
Who taught me this?	
Do I still want it?	
What's a new belief to replace it?	

Core belief	
Who taught me this?	
Do I still want it?	
What's a new belief to replace it?	

Decade Up To Age:

Core belief	
Who taught me this?	
Do I still want it?	
What's a new belief to replace it?	

Core belief	
Who taught me this?	
Do I still want it?	
What's a new belief to replace it?	

Decade Up To Age:

Core belief	
Who taught me this?	
Do I still want it?	
What's a new belief to replace it?	

Core belief	
Who taught me this?	
Do I still want it?	
What's a new belief to replace it?	

Summary for #Women Who Want More

I would like to offer you some thoughts about how to set yourself free and approach this problem from a level of higher energy in order to overcome frustration:

- We may choose to no longer share the same values

- We may choose to no longer share the same beliefs

- We may choose to practice some degree of acceptance of people for who they are, and understand our own power in being us. We don't need to convince anyone but ourselves

- We may choose to understand what may be causing other's behavior, which may be from a place of love or from their own personal frustrations or pain

- We may choose to show compassion for someone who once cared for us who now needs to be cared for. Their role and purpose in life may have changed and this is a difficult thing to come to terms with

- We may choose to redefine our boundaries

- It doesn't actually matter whether the beliefs we come up with are right or wrong; there is no right or wrong—there just is. The main thing is that we make a choice to believe something that makes us feel better about the situation or relationship, and this becomes our truth.

#Insights

Being A Parent

Those of you that are parents know that it's a huge balancing act. It's a balance between being able to guide someone so young, and establishing rapport, respect, and boundaries, while still maintaining good communication, expressing love, being responsible, creating a safe haven within the home, keeping our partners happy, and somehow finding time to do everything. In trying to maintain this balance, we have to try not to lose ourselves in the process. Children grow up and flee the nest someday, at which point there will be questions about how to find yourself again. Your answer to that right now may be "I don't even have time to think about that fact and I'll deal with it when the time comes."

Let me share a story with you about one of my college friends. Let's call her Lucy. Lucy's mother didn't work and when I say she lived her life through her daughter, that even includes the handbags and shoes that she would buy knowing they could be shared. We might have major exams which required hours of study, but Lucy would still be summoned home regardless of that because her mother wanted to celebrate her birthday with her. Naturally, at the same time Lucy was still expected to pass her exams. Lucy has now become a mother herself. She has expressed her fear to me that she is turning into her own mother out of boredom. After having her child, she went back to work for a brief period but then gave that up for several years.

Those first years of motherhood kept Lucy busy and distracted, but as her daughter grew up, she started to question her purpose once again. She started to get depressed, feeling unworthy and undeserving, feeling as if everything she was doing had no value and believing even her daughter didn't value her enough. She tried going back to work part-time even though her family had no need for the money, but she herself had a need for interaction with other people, connection, and purpose. In going back to work she recognized that this didn't answer her needs and she still placed very little value on what she was doing.

In fact, she is very active with fundraising and is full of compassion, always willing to lend an ear, and is one of the most loyal and dear friends anybody could ever wish for. Lucy is an amazing mother, always around to take her daughter to school and extracurricular clubs, spends time with her on holidays, provides nutritious food, and maintains a great family environment. There was no point in my telling her this and expecting her to feel better about herself, though. She needed to figure it out for herself.

In trying to seek fulfillment through being a parent, Lucy was failing. Trying to live her life through her child wasn't giving her purpose and fulfillment. She made sacrifices, but these were not meeting her expectations. What was going to happen when her daughter left home? If we refer back to the previous chapter about leadership, she could have defined her own leadership skills in her parenting, and in so doing, have found more purpose rather than relying on external sources. But it becomes a very fine balancing act when it's not just about you, and you have to consider the needs of young minds as well.

Lucy needed to do the work on herself in order to be energetic and not seek fulfillment from external sources. There was a lot of forgiveness required. Boundaries were a huge issue in that she was quite clearly doing everything to please others but not herself. She was not communicating her needs to the relevant parties in the same way that she hadn't done with her own mother when we were students. She was consumed with guilt about wanting to please herself and interpreted that guilt as meaning perhaps she had failed her daughter in some way by not feeling completely fulfilled in her role of homemaker.

Guilt comes from Level 1 energy and this is the energy that was emanating from her. It is not a level of energy that is productive. If Lucy had been coming from a higher-energy core, she might have seen opportunity, purpose, joy, and thereby received as much love from those around her as she was giving out herself.

As a parent myself, I struggled at one point with my incredible workload while attempting to run a harmonious household, keep my husband happy, keep myself healthy, and at the same time cater to all my children's needs. Those needs encompassed the practicalities of getting them to school, organizing childcare, organizing after-school care and activities, helping with homework and exams, paying for the schools, and those dreaded school projects that we as parents end up doing ourselves. Like any parent, I also needed to show my kids love and receive love, respect them and guide them, nurture them both physically and emotionally, and that's before we even got to simply spend some fun time together.

Talk about juggling! At one stage I quite literally thought the only way to vent my frustration was to scream. I just needed a little bit of space and quiet in order to think clearly, but when you are juggling all that there is no time for quiet. Remember, I have three children, so when two were quiet, inevitably the other one would take advantage of my being free. You may be able to relate to the fact that I couldn't even go to the bathroom in peace. I went to work to get a break and truly admire anyone who looks after their children full-time when they are young.

However, when children get a little bit older you have the chance to communicate on a different level. I started to establish further boundaries. We have a favorite phrase in our household when somebody seems to be taking advantage: "It's not all about you!" My children even use it on me! This phrase encourages the other party or parties to understand that in our family unit we all have to look after each other. If my children drain me and I allow that to happen, what use will I be to them if I'm not well? I could play the martyr and have done so in the past, but how will that serve us in the long-term? What role model will I be for my children if I allow myself to become a victim? Do I want them to imitate that behavior? A great book to read if you're interested in how children take after their parents in non-biological attributes is *Not In Your Genes* by Oliver James.

EXERCISE PATH TO FEELING BETTER
ABOUT OUR PARENTING

Making a Mission Statement

One way of raising the energy levels within the parent/child/family situation is to create a family mission statement. It needs to be one where everyone is involved. I'm not suggesting that your kids put in rules like "no discipline" or "time to play on phones and tablets every night," but a clear vision of how everybody needs to show up within that family unit. The ingredients for the mission statement are as follows (taken from Stephen Covey's *The 7 Habits of Highly Effective Families*—another great resource):

I. Be Proactive – this means responding to the situation based on conscious values and beliefs as opposed to reacting in an emotional way, which is what happens when buttons are pressed due to fear-based values and beliefs. All the parties need to buy in to making this happen and believe that it will and can. If you hear the phrase "nothing will change" or "it's not working out," then the buy-in isn't there. Like everything we've been talking about, you have to make the choice to do it.

II. Begin With The End In Mind – create a clear vision of what your family is all about

III. Prioritize – schedule time with your family to spend together to develop the mission statement

IV. Think Win-Win – this is about resonating at a much higher energy level. It allows a family to realize that every member of the team has a right to win from the situation and compromise doesn't mean that one party pulls one over another. It's very empowering to let everybody know how they will win by establishing a collective vision. They each have a vested interest (buy-in) to make it work. Think for each member: "What's in it for me?"

V. Seek first to understand … and then be understood – this comes down to understanding underlying needs that may not be being communicated. I talked about this in chapter 3 where we touched on understanding needs through nonviolent communication and each person's love language. Taking the time to listen and also ensuring that you are listened to is vital. For example, your child misbehaving may in fact be a cry for help rather than malicious behavior.

VI. Synergize – if each person in the family works together to create something new and is fully bought in to the process, believing that they can make it a reality, then they will feel empowered.

VII. Sharpen the Saw – think about how you and your family could share different physical, social, mental, and spiritual activities together.

The mission statement I developed with my kids is:

That we endeavor to spend fun quality time together and also respect each other's need for privacy. We understand that fulfillment does not only come from family, and that time needs to be allowed for each of us to experience that outside the family unit. We have a need to be responsive to each other as we each grow and develop, and acknowledge that change is the only constant. Effective communication is paramount, and in that, we have a right to express our needs as well as our wants, and have a right to expect them to be met where possible. We all feel love through physical contact (hugs), but understand that that may change and will be communicated effectively and respected. We aim to spend our family time in joint activities, with other family members, with joint friends, and at home relaxing by ourselves in various proportions, to which we will adapt as and when needed. The underlying essence of our family is love. And we don't wake Mummy up in the morning as long as she lets us go to bed later during school holidays!

That last point started when they were young and my good-night ritual with the kids was "Night night, sleep tight, love you, and don't wake me up in the morning!", to which my kids would respond, "I won't, night night, best mummy in the world," and in the interests of outdoing each other as siblings often strive to, this turned into "best mummy to the moon and back; best mummy on the planet; best mummy in the universe!" Bedtime is a loving ritual for us, and as you can see from our mission statement, became an area for negotiation! I still don't get the bathroom to myself, but the collective vision we now share has definitely made life easier, especially in my case where the kids have had to adapt to a divorce and living in two homes.

Our Family Mission Statement

Summary for #Women Who Want More

I would invite you to consider the following when trying to find the balance of parenting and adapting it into your already busy life:

- Consider the role model you are being for your child or children

- Be aware of the beliefs you are passing on to them and the effect that may have on them in later life

- Help them to focus on high-energy positivity (we have a positivity jar at home where the kids write down something positive that happened each day. My daughter calls it a "hap-ment" jar—"happening" and "achievement")

- Help them engage in gratitude – I talked about this previously, and how you can involve kids in that

- Be present and mindful

- Try to hear the kids' needs in their complaints

- Set firm boundaries for yourself emotionally, and for discipline

- Try not to lose yourself and your purpose while bringing up your children

- Guilt is a wasted use of energy

- If you don't look after yourself, what kind of parent or partner can you be?

- Communicate your needs as clearly as you can and respect others'

- The best way to show love is to be love

- Create a high-energy but calm home environment and see time as abundant

- Share responsibility among all of you

- Prioritize your values as they relate to parenting, and allow yourself to express them. If some are low priority, then consider letting them go and not worrying too much

- Create a family vision and adapt it accordingly

- When someone tells you how amazing you are, or that you're "super-mum"—accept the compliment graciously and say, "I know!" because you deserve the compliment and believe that you can only do what you can, and only be who you are

#Insights

Yet To Become A Parent

If you haven't encountered difficulty in conceiving, but know that you will want children, then establishing expectations beforehand can prove very helpful. Consider creating your family mission statement from the outset. Reflect on all aspects of your life and how you might maintain the balance. Set your boundaries and create limits. Be clear on your values and how you will honor them as a parent. Define your purpose, and how you might draw from all aspects of your life to establish that. Hopefully the previous section about parenthood equating to survival didn't put you off!

A lot of us automatically want to become parents because it's just the norm, and we think there must be something wrong with us if we don't. There is nothing right or wrong, normal or abnormal with either decision—it just is. My sister didn't want children and was adamant about it for the first seven years of her marriage until some instinct kicked in and she then found herself unable to conceive naturally and needed IVF treatment.

I shared a little of my story with you, where I had five miscarriages, and so strong was the need in me to have a third child that I risked my own life and went against medical advice in order to carry my now beautiful seven-year-old boy. I cannot explain to you the overwhelming sense of fulfillment I felt when he was born, and the gratitude to my husband for creating him with me, in the same way I cannot verbalize the excruciating pain and sorrow of flushing my first miscarried child (at 12 weeks) down a toilet while on holiday in Greece, and going through the physical pain of labor while delivering a child I already knew to be dead and then proceeding to have to bury him on my own. My milk came in after that, only to add to the emotional turmoil. I was back at work, caring for patients and smiling on the outside, the next day.

So how, if you so desperately want children, can you remain calm about it? That's what you're supposed to do in order to conceive, right? Easier said than done, of course. One client of mine shared her story with me.

I'll refer to her as Jenny. For years Jenny had gone through every possible treatment in an attempt to conceive. This had placed so much stress on her relationship that it broke down, and putting that together with turning 40 and her biological clock ticking was potentially too much to bear. As years went on, she became a foster mother, thinking that that would feed her need. Sadly, that only lasted a year or so during which she gave her all to the girls who were placed in her care, leaving her feeling completely drained and unwell. No other relationship worked out, which in her words was "because I always pick people who have something wrong with them," and she couldn't face fostering again for fear of repeating the experience where she had given herself completely, only to receive very little in return. To add to the tragedy, Jenny had previously worked as a nanny and so there was no way she wanted to open the wounds of not being able to have children by spending all day looking after someone else's kids. On the surface, she presented herself as a smiling, charming, attractive woman.

She had defined her purpose in life as being a mother, and was stuck, unable to think of any other way to fulfill that purpose. She would get angry about what had happened to her, and then retreat back. She had traveled so far down the line of just wanting this one thing that she believed would give her life meaning that she forgot to live in the now. She forgot to be present or to care for her emotional, mental, and physical health. She forgot to care for her relationship and identify her needs and boundaries. Jenny was so focused on having kids that she stopped having fun. Yes, she wanted a child, but what was it she believed that child would give her?

Therein lies the clue. She had two foster children, but it wasn't what she was expecting. What Jenny actually needed, her purpose in life if you will, was love. And everywhere she looked for it—in children, in relationships, from her parents—it was missing. But she wasn't really looking in the right place because if she had looked within herself, she would have seen that she needed to start by loving herself. By doing just that, her energy could evolve from being a victim (Level 1)into one of love, purpose, and joy (levels 4,5 and 6). Of course, she needed to believe that she deserved it first.

Notice how we keep ending up at the same point in all of these stories: the essence is exploring who you are, and needing to shift how you show up so that your reality in turn will shift around you.

While this is a sad story, I use it here as an illustration of the importance of maintaining balance in your life. Don't focus on one thing you think will make you happy and let everything else fall by the wayside. What if that thing doesn't happen? What then? I was fortunate enough to feel that fulfillment after having my children, but it only lasted for a limited period until I started searching for the next thing to add to it.

EXERCISE PATH TO HAPPY PARENTING

I'm not sure you can ever be ready for parenthood and all its joys and stresses. However, making a rule book with your partner can be a fun, creative exercise to do.

Making Your Parenting Rule Book

- The first set of rules should be about each of your hopes in turn – what each of you hopes to get out of it individually

- The next set should work out some joint expectations – this might be that you both hope to be able to spend more time together as a family unit, or perhaps you want to redefine your quality time as a couple

- Next, start to list the possible challenges that may come up and how you might overcome them. This might be financial, work- or health-related, or possibly even the inability to conceive and how you will choose to deal and cope should that happen. If you're stuck for ideas – just ask any parents, I'm sure they'll make some suggestions

- Next, make a promise to yourself. This needs to be a powerful statement to help you overcome the biggest fear you may have. So for example, if you fear that you will gain weight and never fit into your skinny jeans again then bringing this fear to the surface empowers you to promise yourself that you won't allow that to happen. If your fear is that you will lose your identity, then promise yourself otherwise. If you fear that you may not cope, then make a bold statement to yourself about the fact that you will cope easily and be brilliant!

Parental Rule Book

You may wish to jot down some thoughts about what you'd like to list in your rule book including:

Your hopes

Joint expectations

Potential challenges and solutions

Powerful intentions

Summary for #Women Who Want More

I'd invite you to consider the following if you have a future desire to add to your family with children:

- o Be true to yourself at all times

- o Define your purpose and how it can be fulfilled

- o Find balance in all aspects of your life, avoiding making just one thing the focus

- o Set your boundaries

- o Be clear on your expectations

- o Give gratitude

- o Ask for help

- o Communicate well

- o Express your needs

- o Try to have fun!

#Insights

CHAPTER 6

KEEPING EVERYBODY HAPPY –
OUR FRIENDS, OUR PARTNERS, OUR FAMILIES

*"Everything that irritates us about others can lead us to an
understanding of ourselves."*
~ Carl Jung

What do we want from a relationship? What does it give us? How do we
show up in it? What characteristics are important to us in the people we
form relationships with? What patterns keep repeating themselves?

I'd like to start this chapter with one of the foundational principles
introduced to me by my coaching school (iPEC), as I think it
encompasses so many of the answers to these questions.

"Each person we meet is our teacher and student."

What we are talking about here is connection. As much as we may play
the helper in a relationship, there is always an opportunity to also learn

from the other person. I learn as much from my children, friends, and clients as they do from me. Conversely, if you have always been looked after, then you are teaching the person looking after you about themselves.

There may be friendships or partners that come and go, but in considering that they were not chance meetings or mistakes, and actually were opportunities to learn, what did you learn from them? As harsh as it may sound, just like beliefs, certain people may no longer serve you as you grow and evolve.

In a previous chapter I discussed issues with parents, and how our values and beliefs may differ from theirs as we form our own conscious-based ones through our own experiences. The same applies to every relationship we have, be it a friend, partner, family member, or colleague.

I recall doing a values exercise with my coach shortly after my divorce. I remember when I first signed up for her program and the warm fuzzy feeling that washed over me when she said we would start with finding out just who Rana was. I realized then that I actually had no idea. After the exercise in which we identified my values, she asked me to be aware over the coming weeks of the people around me and the emotions they evoked.

Selfishness was one of the characteristics I had no tolerance for, and yet I realized I had been married to someone who exhibited that trait so strongly, where I showed none of it. In fact, having now established boundaries, I recognize that a degree of selfishness is important, but it was an example of why my relationship with my husband was so imbalanced. One value I found incredibly important was respect, and I started to recognize that I had felt very disrespected in my marriage. Conversely, I had felt respected in my working relationships and by my friends, so I felt more myself and seen in those relationships.

Once I identified what was in me, I started to stand in that power, and noticed how I attracted more people who shared my values, and how those who didn't started to fall by the wayside. For those relationships that I didn't want to lose but which grated at times, such as family members, recognizing the difference in values allowed me to be more accepting. It gave me the opportunity to release catabolic energy, and allowed me to move forward without emotional button pushing.

We talked in previous chapters about the need for boundaries and how to set them. It's important to apply these boundaries to all relationships. I'll give you an example of a boundary I had to redefine with one of my closest friends. We now both have children and so we don't get to see as much of each other as we used to, what with juggling our children's personal calendars and the chauffeuring that entails, plus work commitments. I'm sure some of you can relate. For me, if I set a confirmed date in my diary to meet, then that time is sacred. It means I won't cancel if something else comes along. I am fully committed and unless an unforeseen circumstance emerges, I'll be there.

My friend, on the other hand, was forever canceling on me at the last minute. There was always a valid excuse, but it was clear her priorities were not the same as mine. I used to get so frustrated and feel disrespected, as though she was making a statement that my time was not valued, that her other friends or family were more important than me, and she was now wasting my precious time. I got quite worked up about it and made up all these stories in my head which further fueled my frustration.

As I became more communicative about my needs, I brought the conversation to the table. She hadn't realized all the other commitments I might have turned down when setting a date to spend time with her. She hadn't realized that canceling a last-minute weekend event meant that my children's plans were also compromised because I might have turned down parties they could have otherwise gone to. She hadn't fully appreciated that I was feeling disrespected by all this. In having this conversation with her, I expressed my understanding that I knew how important her family was to her and how difficult she found it to let them down. She found it easier to let me down because she knew I would understand better than they would. When you look at things another way, it's actually a compliment that she trusted me enough not to turn on her where others might have.

During the conversation I expressed how her behavior was making me feel and also expressed what my needs were and where my boundaries lay. Recognizing what buttons were being pressed, and the stories I was telling myself through her behavior allowed us to clear the air. In her case she still has much work to do when it comes to setting boundaries in her own life, but we know that in our friendship, we are both coming from a place of love and acceptance. Has her behavior changed? No. Do I feel better about the situation? Yes. I got it off my chest, I felt heard and understood, and I made a conscious choice not to judge her for the choices she makes, and to feel differently about the situation in the future. I released catabolic energy and raised my energy to a more anabolic one.

I'm sure most of us can think of situations that may relate to relationships and to feeling annoyed when people don't respond to text messages. WhatsApp is the worst for that because you can see when someone has actually read or listened to your message and then you wonder why on earth they haven't responded to you yet. I've altered my privacy settings so that no one can see when I was last online or if I've read a message because I don't want them to get annoyed with me. There is always a good reason why I may not have responded. Whether or not they understand that depends on their own beliefs and interpretations. The privacy settings give me freedom not to have to explain myself. Not to feel guilty. They give me a kind of power.

I'll share another example here of one of my clients. I'll call her Rebecca. Rebecca was somebody who needed to be super organized and liked to plan everything in advance. She would chase assignments and try to get clear on the expectations placed on her with plenty of time to spare so that she could plan and execute accordingly. Her business partner, however, was much more relaxed about things. Here we have a case of my client telling herself that her business partner didn't respect her and at the same time feeling very out of control because she needed the information in order to live her life calmly. She got very emotional about it, feeling anger, frustration, and powerlessness. Rebecca's business partner, on the other hand, didn't feel his behavior was disrespectful. He didn't recognize that Rebecca might be planning to complete an assignment one month ahead of time and therefore needed information sent to her early.

I asked Rebecca what another interpretation might look like and what her business partner might be thinking. Helping her to express her needs as well as her wants when making her requests helped to re-establish a healthier and more balanced and energetic relationship. It gave her a sense of power back.

How does the relationship serve you?

So far we have talked about values, beliefs, boundaries, communication, and interpretations. Let's take this a step further and talk about what's in it for you. We receive different things from different people. Among other things, I receive unconditional love from my children, appreciation from my partner, respect from my work colleagues, and admiration from my friends.

I also play different roles in those relationships. With my children, I am the carer and provider; with my partner, I am the equal; with my friends, I am the listener; with my work colleagues, I am the leader.

The relationships that are strong and which have served me well are those that meet my needs, albeit in different proportions. The challenge in a family or intimate relationship is that you hope to grow together and that as your needs evolve, they will continue to be met. However, we often look back with regret at relationships that may have ended, and frequently play either the victim or feel guilty about how we may have treated the other person.

There was once a very strong pattern in my life of giving endlessly in an abusive relationship until there was nothing left to give and because I didn't receive what I needed, I would get incredibly drained and then eventually find the strength to end the relationship. Even so, I would still lament the good qualities that that person had and wonder if maybe I had tried harder or expressed myself differently it might have worked out after all. I would continue to blame myself and in so doing, continue the story that I had allowed myself to feel in the relationship— one of unworthiness, un-deservedness, and regret. These are all feelings fueled by catabolic energy.

After my divorce and in finding myself, I still fell into some of these types of relationships. However, I'm pleased to say that they didn't last very long. I no longer allowed them to because I had started to stand into my own power. Did I feel lonely? Of course I did, but I recognized that I was lonelier in a relationship that didn't meet my needs than not being in a relationship at all. Each time one of these relationships would end I made it a habit of writing down exactly how that relationship hadn't met my needs. Just reading my notes back to myself gave me the complete power to be me again. It gave me the power to be one of those people who was quite happy to delete the phone number, email address, and all the previous text messages and communications we might have had.

I did the same thing with some of my friendships after my divorce. Understandably, people feel awkward in these kinds of situations and you have expectations of your friends. You may interpret their behavior as disloyal and be blind to the love they may be trying to show you. I didn't want our joint friends to take sides and fortunately for me those friends that counted have been able to continue relationships with both of us.

For those that fell by the wayside, I was able to let go in the knowledge that they no longer served me. One of those was a very close friendship I had had for over 10 years. Our firstborns had grown up together and she was one of those people who would defend me if I was ever wronged in some way. She was loyal and supportive in my darkest moments. However, after my divorce, perhaps my life wasn't quite as turbulent and I didn't have as much to complain about. I started to stand into my power and so her role needed to change. In a headspace of peace and resolution, I started to resent the anger and judgments that she would place on anything I had to say.

My needs changed from having someone voicing indignation on my behalf to needing someone who could care for me in a different way. It broke my heart when we finally parted ways. However, I only need to recall how I stood before her crying and she literally turned her back on me to remind myself how that relationship was no longer serving me. I didn't need to justify my actions and not feel understood as I had in my marriage. No doubt she must have had other things going on in her life that led her to feel anger towards me. I must have triggered something and she undoubtedly told herself a story very different to mine.

I'm not suggesting we turn our backs on every friendship but I am trying to illustrate the power you give yourself when you let go of those relationships that no longer serve you. It not only gives you power but also space. Space to be the person you have become and space to let new people into your life.

So how do you show up in a relationship?

How well do your family members, work friends, college friends, school friends, friends from your kids' schools, etc., mix? Do you actually try to bring them together? I recall one of my patients deciding to have a fiftieth year celebration during which she celebrated her fiftieth birthday every month of that year, each time with a different group of friends instead of one big fiftieth birthday party. There can be advantages to having different groups of friends that don't interact! However, have you ever asked yourself why those friends don't mix? Why should other people like each other because you like them and they like you? That leads to awkwardness with you trying to keep everybody happy and not having such a great time. Well, if you haven't figured it out already, you're trying to be a different person with each set of people.

Historically my work colleagues have seen me as quiet, studious, and professional; my college friends as dynamic, organized, and fun. My family may have seen me as bossy, driven, and exceptional; my school friends as wacky and fun; my children as loving and compassionate. Not surprisingly, I am all of those things and a great deal more, but I wear different hats in different surroundings. Consider how you are showing up in any relationship and what proportion of yourself you are showing to others.

I think of myself as kind, loving, compassionate, sensitive, intuitive, dynamic, fun, crazy, and vibrant, to name a few. Why can't everybody see that? It was only in growing as a person, and becoming more conscious, that I started to see synergy in the people around me. I never used to show my spiritual side to my family, for example, for fear they would think I was completely mad. I would hide my sensitive side at work and wonder why they didn't show compassion when I was hurting so much inside. How were they supposed to know if I didn't show them? There is a need here to be brave enough to expose your vulnerability. A need to take off the mask, which you may not be able to do in a work situation, but is well worth the rewards in an intimate relationship. If you do it and your needs are not met, then what's the worst that can happen? You always have a choice. You always have power.

When I fell in love with my partner, it was the most unique relationship I had ever experienced because for the first time in my life I felt truly seen. He had no expectations of me. He saw my vulnerability and my need to be loved and he honored that. It only happened because I took off the mask with him and then also with so many friends. Now I'm in a situation where I would quite happily bring together the friends I have made in the last five years and feel confident that they have a lot more in common than just being my friend. They are like-minded individuals who share so many of the same values, beliefs, and characteristics, and we have a mutual respect for each other's needs.

EXERCISE PATH TO HAVING BALANCED ENERGETIC RELATIONSHIPS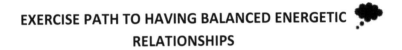

Here are two exercises you can try based on what we've discussed so far. Download the worksheets from www.lightchangescoaching.com.

1- Creating Your Energetic Relationship

The first exercise is about finding the ideal partner or if you already have one, then deepening that relationship by understanding it further. Draw two columns. In the first column, list what characteristics you want your ideal partner to have. This can be anything at all, even what they look like. There is no need to feel embarrassed about that aspect if it's important to you. If you don't write things down because you're embarrassed then you're telling the universe that you're embarrassed and don't really want those qualities in a partner.

In the next column say how each characteristic meets your needs or what value that is important to you it represents. If you have a partner, draw a third column. In that column, grade from a scale of 1 to 10, where 10 is the most, how often that need is being met, or a value is being honored. Of course, you can also do this exercise based on a friendship or family member.

I'll give you some examples here to help you along. If you want your ideal partner to be emotionally intelligent, this may represent your need for understanding; if you want your partner to be adventurous, this may represent how you value fun and enjoyment or freedom, and the need for that to be honored. If you want your partner to be financially stable, then this may be a desire to meet your needs for financial stability or possibly represent the value you place on abundance.

Creating Your Energetic Relationship

Relationship:

List What You Want From The Person In This Relationship	What Need Or Value Does This Fulfil In You	How Often Does It Show Up (Scale 1-10)

I wanted my partner to have a healthy diet and not to be overweight. For me, that wasn't just to do with appearance but it represented my value of healthy living. Someone who was overweight represented somebody who might not respect that value. I have shared with you how highly I place respect on my value list. Of course, that's my interpretation of what I see and we all have different stories.

One of my clients used this exercise to stop herself from going back to her long-term partner who she knew in her heart wasn't right for her and it also stopped her from pursuing ones that were never likely to meet her needs. She became empowered.

Go all out with this exercise. Play with it, be creative with it, and don't hold anything back if it's something you truly want and need. If you apply a scoring system and find that something is lacking in your relationship, then that may be an area of discussion for you to have with your partner or friend based on expressing your needs as well as your wants, which is the foundation of nonviolent communication.

2- How Am I Seen?

This next exercise will help you to reflect on how you are showing up. Draw five columns and title them strangers, work colleague(s), friend(s), partner (this may be present or past), family member(s) (again, you may want to separate these out). In each column, list at least three characteristics of how that person is likely to see you.

How Am I Seen?

Strangers	Work Colleagues	Friends	Partner	Family Members

How different are the characteristics in each column? Do the characteristics actually represent the same thing but in different words? If so, why?

This exercise is a great way of putting down on paper how you are showing up in each type of relationship in your life. We have talked about the freedom of being your authentic self and so the more you evolve and understand about yourself, the more you grow, the more conscious you become, the more you will find that the similarities in these columns resemble each other until you will hopefully be using the same words. It's a reflective exercise, so ask yourself questions as to why you have listed different things in each column. If it doesn't bother you, then you don't need to do anything about it. But there may well be clues as to why, when you consider relationships in which you feel happy and fulfilled, as opposed to ones where you may be feeling misunderstood or unseen.

A high-energy relationship will have a balanced amount of communication, mutual support, boundaries, trust, friendship, intimacy, and honesty. On that note, I'd like to end this chapter with an excerpt from the poem, "The Dance," taken from Oriah Mountain Dreamer's book, *The Dance*.

Take me to the places on the earth that teach you how to dance, the places where you can risk letting the world break your heart.

And I will take you to the places where the earth beneath my feet and the stars overhead make my heart whole again and again.

Summary for #Women Who Want More

I invite you to consider the following points as they relate to relationships:

- There is no need for regrets. Everything is a learning opportunity

- Why do patterns keep repeating themselves? What is it that you need to learn in order to set yourself free?

- Are your values being honored in the relationship?

- What other interpretation could you form about the situation or person?

- Nobody makes us feel a certain way. We gain power by recognizing that we have chosen to feel that way

- We may not be able to change the people or situation, but we can change how we feel about it

- Be clear on what it is you need from a relationship

- How are your needs being met?

- Be honest and true to yourself

- How is the relationship serving you?

- How are you showing up in a relationship? Are you wearing a mask?

- Have you set boundaries and are you honoring them?

- What love language do you and your partner each speak? (referred to in chapter 2)

- How can you improve your communication to get what you need?

- It's okay to let go of things or people that no longer serve you

- In vulnerability, there is power

#Insights

CHAPTER 7

I SHOULD REALLY EXERCISE AND EAT HEALTHILY ...

"Food is not just fuel. Food is about family, food is about community, food is about identity. And we nourish all those things when we eat well."
~ Michael Pollan

What is your relationship with food? Where does it stem from? How much exercise do you get? Why do you exercise? How much do you love your body?

Our relationship with food can be a complex one. On the one hand, we need it to give us energy and keep us alive, while on the other we may hate what it has the potential to do to us. We can gain so much pleasure from eating the "wrong" foods, only to be wracked with guilt afterwards. We can allow it to control us, rather than us controlling it.

Food, nutrition, and exercise are areas in our lives where we struggle by telling ourselves that we should, but do not. This state of "should" resonates at a low-energy frequency because we're not giving ourselves power and choice. How many times have you vowed to make it back to the gym and go every week? How many times have you vowed never to consume the whole tub of Ben & Jerry's? How many times have you made New Year's resolutions to change your eating or exercise regimes only to forget by the time you get to February? How many times have you done the new fad diet, only for your weight to spiral back up again?

Not surprisingly, a great deal of this starts with the beliefs that we adopt as children. I have shared with you already the opinions of my relatives who called me fat. I got so sick of hearing it, and obviously thought it was true, that I stopped taking my lunch money to school so I had no option but to go hungry.

I shared a room with my sister growing up, and envied her flat stomach. I was in joyous shock when I woke up one morning and saw my own flat stomach reflecting back at me. Did it make me happy? Of course it did, but I couldn't possibly ruin it, so I then proceeded to avoid eating. As I got older, I discovered how laxatives allowed me to eat what I wanted, and I could then purge myself. I found solace with one of my friends who was quite clearly the same and we would be consumed with tragic, hysterical laughter about the trips she made to the pharmacy asking for laxatives as if they were drugs, or feeling so desperate when she ran out of her stash that she would try drinking pints of saltwater in the hope it would have the same effect. I am laughing now as I write this because it really was quite funny, albeit tragically so.

Bulimia typically affects those who have been through stressful transitions or life changes, have a history of abuse or trauma, negative body image, or poor self-esteem—all of which I had. I would ravage a packet of biscuits, only to then dose up on laxatives or engage in hours of exercise. I needed to have control, and that was my way of controlling the situation. I was obsessed about my relationship with food; what I had eaten in a day would control my life, such was the imbalance. Exercise was my way of dealing with emotions I couldn't face. You couldn't get me out of the gym after my mother died. I needed to feel better and that was how I did it – through distraction and alternative pain.

I still battle with my relationship with food and exercise today, but have mostly managed to shift into a mindset where it no longer controls me. I have found balance. How did I do it? Well, we talked earlier about the need for love and forgiveness, which is something I certainly needed to do. I also needed to go deeper in exploring my values and beliefs and choosing new ones. I learned to control the situation rather than allowing it to control me. I gave myself permission to view food and exercise in different ways, concentrating on the benefits they could have rather than the punishments they inflicted upon me. I transitioned from an imbalance of obsessing over food and exercise to the detriment of other aspects of my life, into one where each component of my life had significance and purpose and could give me an element of fulfillment and control. I shifted from making fear-based choices to conscious-based move-toward choices. Let me explain that a little more for you.

A fear-based choice might be something like exercising three times a week because you're worried that you might get cellulite. A more conscious-based choice is deciding to exercise three times a week because you believe that it will keep you healthy. Can you see the difference? In the first example you had a fear of developing cellulite. Now, if you are carrying that fear with you, then you are resonating from a lower energy level. The latter is a more powerful choice, resonating at a higher energy level because it has nothing to do with fear and what might happen to you; it's about the opportunity the action offers you.

You may hear references to being a carrot or stick person. This refers to a rabbit that runs away from the stick (fear), or towards the carrot (the desire). Different beliefs motivate different people, which is a strong argument for why we can't tell people what to do. What is important and a priority for one of us is not necessarily the case for someone else, and the same advice will not work for everyone. It is far more powerful for you yourself to come up with the actions you want to take, which is something we help you with in core-energy™ coaching.

Let's go back to the two people starting out on an exercise regimen and see how that applies. One (person A) has a motivation to lose weight, so not surprisingly, once they reach their target weight, their motivation is gone and so they don't continue with the program. The other person (B) may have chosen to exercise because they wanted to have more energy every day. They may have recognized that if they stopped exercising, then their energy levels would drop again. Person B's motivation to continue exercising is very different, and it will be pointless encouraging them to stand on the scales as that is not relevant to them. They may maintain the exercise regimen for longer because their motivation is coming from a deeper level of desire than reaching a target weight. I would encourage you to consider this when you buy a book or generalized program that makes promises about weight loss or how to achieve the perfect body.

There's a great chapter in the book *The Secret* by Rhonda Byrne where she talks about her relationship with food. She shifted her belief system from one where she thought if she ate the wrong foods she would put on weight, to a belief system where she viewed everything she ate as nutritious and wholesome and with love. She shifted her belief system to one where she believed she could eat anything she wanted, it would nourish her body, and she would not gain weight. She found that it worked for her and she can now eat anything she likes. The power of the mind is truly astounding.

Have you looked at people who seem to get away with eating anything they want and envied them? Yes, I can give you the scientific explanation of their rapid metabolism, but it is also very likely that they don't even think very much about what and when they are eating, and it's likely they also don't worry about it. They may have always been like that, in which case why would they worry? Most of us, however, need to shift our beliefs because it is not something we have known for our whole lives.

The classic example here may be the limiting belief that we gain weight when we hit our forties and go through menopause. It's understandable that we have that belief; it's in all the literature, all the images we see, and is what we hear from our parents or friends. How freeing would it be to choose not to have that belief? If you tell yourself that is what is going to happen—guess what? It most likely will! Because the energy you resonate will influence that. You will be resonating from Level 1 where something is happening to you without any control. And as you gain weight, you will be compounding the evidence even further, and feel powerless to change it. A higher-energy way to consider it may be from a place of gratitude, or fearlessness, where you choose to be grateful for the ability to still eat as you have always done and are fearless about the changes in hormones that are affecting your body.

As a scientist, one of my areas of research was on the effect of stress on our ability to recover from chronic illness. The power of the human brain is limitless. I'll talk more about that when we come to health in the next chapter, but please note that there is no replacement for good medical advice. If your weight is fluctuating disproportionately to your habits, then please seek medical advice—there could be a sound reason.

EXERCISE PATH TO TURNING 'SHOULD' INTO 'WANT'

We've talked about fears, beliefs, and motivating factors so far. So how can you discover what your deepest motivation is in order to maintain sustainable results? This is where I joke about 'man-flu' and how it can only be real flu if you can't bring yourself to get out of bed to get to the bottom of the garden to retrieve the £50 note.

What is it that is going to make you get out of bed on a cold rainy morning and go to the gym? What is that, no matter how much the little voice in your head is giving you every excuse possible to avoid, will be a louder voice that makes you go anyway?

What is it that is going to make you choose a healthy salad over a burger and fries from the menu? What will make you pass on that second glass of wine? What will stop you from opening the freezer door and taking out the whole tub of ice cream instead of just a few scoops?

Shall we find out? I like to call this exercise "Peeling the Onion." I adapted it from Dean Graziosi's "Seven-Levels Deep" in his book *Millionaire Success Habits: The Gateway to Wealth & Prosperity*, a recommended read.

It's a little like having a seven-year-old child. Do you start to get really annoyed because they keep asking why? Each time you give them an answer, they ask why again. And why? And why? Until you run out of answers or patience and tell them to be quiet! Well, that is exactly what we're going to do in this exercise. I'll talk you through it and then use an example to help you along.

It's a good idea to clear your mind thoroughly before doing this exercise, so take the opportunity to sit quietly and breathe for a few minutes or use the centering exercise that I mentioned you can download from www.lightchangescoaching.com. I'd also recommend downloading the worksheet for this exercise at the same time.

Peeling The Onion

The first thing to do is consider a goal you want to achieve. In this chapter we've been talking about diet and exercise so let's use an example such as wanting to exercise for five hours a week. Write that goal down at the top of the worksheet. Then, in the first box, write down the question "Why do you want to exercise five hours a week?" In the box next to it, write your answer. It should be the first thing that springs to mind, which is why centering yourself beforehand is really useful to clear your head.

Once you have your answer, ask why you want to do that. Write it down in the same way in the next row on the worksheet. An answer to that question might be, "I want to exercise for five hours a week because I've been told to." In the box in the second row you would then write, "Why have you been told to exercise for five hours a week?" and then you would write your answer in the box next to it. Keep on repeating this process until you have asked that question so many times that you feel totally stuck on an answer—then give it one final push and ask it one more time.

What you are effectively doing as you peel away these layers of the onion is shifting from your head into your heart. You are transitioning from "should" and the story you tell yourself, to "want" and a desire within you that needs to be fulfilled. It takes at least three initial layers to move from head to heart and by the time you get to a sixth layer you may well have the answer of what your deepest motivation may be and what's going to help you to achieve whatever goal you have to set. By the time you get to the last layer, just like peeling an onion is painful to your eyes and can generate tears, this exercise may do the same. That's perfectly okay!!

I'll follow the whole process through for you to see how this works. I did want to exercise for five hours a week. Now in my case, exercise is not something I find particularly difficult because I happen to really love working out and in fact was a fitness instructor alongside being a dentist for over 10 years. Of course, now I have a busy career, one where I frequently travel and have no regular pattern where I can allocate every Saturday morning to going to the gym because I might be in a hotel in another country and I have children with commitments that could impact my time to exercise. So what will ensure that I do five hours of exercise a week wherever I happen to be and whatever my schedule looks like? And how will I find that time if it isn't a regular time?

My first response is because I have been told to exercise five hours a week.

Why have you been told?

Because my doctor told me it is good for me.

Why did your doctor tell you it is good for you?

Because he said it would reduce my risk of breast cancer.

Why do you want to exercise for five hours a week to avoid breast cancer?

Because that's how my mother died.

Why is exercising five hours a week important to come to terms with how your mother died?

I don't want to die the same way.

Why don't you want to die the same way?

It's not that I'm scared of dying, but I'm not ready to die anytime soon.

Why are you not ready to die anytime soon?

Because I want to be around to see my children grow up. I don't want them to feel as lost as I did when my mother died. I want to show them love and be loved by them and be present for as long as I possibly can.

Why is that the case?

Because they need me and I need them.

That final answer is what drags me out of my hotel bed and forces me to make sure I exercise even when there isn't a gym. You can see how this shift has occurred from being told to do something and being advised that it's good for me, to what my deepest motivation is. I think of that motivating factor when I'm really struggling to get myself going. *It is E-*

motive, as in *emotionally* motivating and *energetically* motivating. I have my E-Motive written down and take that piece of paper with me when I travel so that I can remember. I share the motivation with my kids so they end up holding me accountable and make sure I fit my exercise into the week.

This is an easy exercise to do either on your own or, even more powerfully, with somebody else because they will hold the space for you and help to push deeper as you eventually peel off all the layers and see the core inside. I know I'm using this exercise as it relates to food and lifestyle, but you can use it with any goal in your life when you question your deeper motivation. Consider sharing your deepest final answer and placing it somewhere visible so you can refer to it and help keep yourself motivated.

Peeling The Onion

What is the goal?

Why?

Why?

Why?

Why?

Why?

Why?

Why?

Why?

My E-Motive to:

Is:

A final word on behavior change and the process that occurs. I learned this 'stages of change model' back in medical school and used it with my patients for years when trying to instigate behavioral change. When we think about making a change, typically it is triggered by an event that shifts us from precontemplation into contemplation. This might be a relative dying from a heart attack and so you start thinking about quitting smoking. You then find an inner motivating factor (determination), put it into action, and at any stage may well relapse and then carry on for a while with the relapsed behavior (in this case smoking again) until you choose to enter the cycle again, usually due to something else happening to give you a nudge.

Sticking with the smoking example, people usually try to quit at least three times and relapse before managing to give up permanently. I hope that by using the peeling the onion exercise you can imagine how the transition from contemplation to determination phase can potentially become much more deeply embedded. As a coach, I take my clients past that step into action plans and accountability to help them stay in the cycle rather than fall off the wagon.

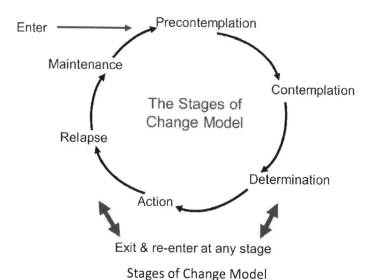

Stages of Change Model

Summary for #Women Who Want More

I invite you to consider some of the following when trying to find balance in your nutrition and exercise choices.

- What is your relationship with food?

- How do you feel about food?

- How do you feel about exercise?

- What are the beliefs you grew up with?

- How well do those beliefs serve you now?

- How in control do you feel about nutrition and exercise?

- What is the story you tell yourself?

- What might be a more powerful story and belief you could choose?

- How much love do you give yourself?

- What are your goals around diet and exercise?

- Where do those goals stem from? (What need?)

- What are the energetic influencers that might be getting in the way? (spiritual, mental, emotional, physical, social, environmental – as described in Ch. 1)

#Insights

CHAPTER 8

PERFECT HEALTH AND EXUBERANT ENERGY – IS IT EVEN POSSIBLE?

"It is health that is real wealth and not pieces of gold and silver."
~ Mahatma Gandhi

What does perfect health mean to you? How much emphasis do you put on it? What self-care behaviors do you engage in? How do you feel about getting older? How much support do you have? How much energy do you have?

I recall going on my first hiking trip to Thailand in 2000. There was a 70-year-old in the group. That was positively ancient to a then-20-something. He was fitter than all of us, slim, muscled, and exuded vitality. My perception at the time was that he must surely be the exception—70 was old!!!! I now look at myself aged 45, and am a far cry from where my mother was at my age. I am slimmer, far more active, more flexible, more energetic, and engage in far more self-care. Using my new beliefs, I have superseded the old belief that a 45-year-old can't be that way.

When I ask my patients about their medical history and then ask them why they have high blood pressure, or diabetes, or why they are on medication for high cholesterol, or why their thyroid is underactive, the most frequent answers I get back are either "It's age—I'm getting old" or "I don't know."

If you've stayed with me to this point in the book then you'll know what I'm getting at and start to recognize patterns. Somebody just taking medication and not fully understanding why they are taking it, but surrendering themselves into the hands of a doctor, is Level 1 energy. They're in victim mode and are completely allowing somebody else to look after them. Of course, this level of energy has exactly that advantage—that *they* don't have to do anything and people will look after them. But where is the power in that? How can they get better if they don't understand why they are unwell in the first place and take ownership of their condition?

When I was a child growing up, my dad used to comment on how we were so lucky that we might not have very much money, but we all had our health. As a teenager, that meant nothing to me. I had no concept of what the importance of health was. That is hardly surprising given that I hadn't actually experienced ill health either firsthand or around anybody in my family. How many times do you hear of someone dying and at that moment in time acknowledge how life is just too short and you have to make the most of every moment?

Naturally, it's human nature to forget those promises and then just sink back into old patterns of being busy, preoccupied, and juggling daily life, forgetting to make the most of every moment. We take our health for granted until something goes wrong. Have you ever suffered a knee sprain and only then recognized how much you enjoyed walking in the woods because that luxury was taken away from you? What effect does finding yourself unable to enjoy life as you once did have on your mental and emotional state? And in turn what does that mental state then have on your physical health?

I touched earlier on the effect of stress on chronic illnesses. It can have an indirect effect in that when you are experiencing stress, you no longer engage in health-positive behaviors. That might mean you drink more alcohol, smoke more, and eat unhealthily. It also has a direct effect on our immune systems and organs function. Cortisol levels and hormonal imbalances contribute to weight gain, organ malfunction, skin disorders, irregularities in menstruation, and infertility, to name but a few. You hear of people dying from a broken heart, particularly when couples who have been together for so long lose their partner and end up following shortly afterwards. Yes, they may suddenly die of a heart attack or cancer, but how has it come on so quickly? It is the mental and emotional state that has created the biological response in their body and led to a physical manifestation of illness.

Louise Hay's story is one of incredible inspiration. She was diagnosed with incurable cancer. She took responsibility for her own healing and within six months of ridding herself of all the emotional baggage she had been carrying with her since childhood, and choosing new thoughts, beliefs, and behavior patterns, the doctors confirmed that she no longer had any trace of cancer in her body. Right up until her recent death, Hay was an advocate for personal growth and development and espoused the belief that if you are willing to change the way you think, believe, and act, then you can have anything you want in life. Her international bestseller, *You Can Heal Your Life*, is an inspirational read and includes parts of her small book *Heal Your Body*, in which she lists every illness, the probable mental and emotional cause that leads to that physical manifestation, and what new thought pattern can help overcome that physical condition. To use the phrase "the proof is in the pudding," Hay certainly led by example.

If we consider the law of attraction where anything we think about repeatedly manifests, then focusing on what we don't want can manifest just that into our lives. I have known people to spend so much time worrying about getting cancer that sure enough, that's exactly what happened. In cases like these, where the emphasis is tipped so heavily towards health and imbalanced with other aspects of life, we can bring illness into our lives—the exact thing we have been trying to avoid. It is so important to shift your energetic focus from fear-based and what you don't want, to what is it you do want. So as we are talking about health, instead of thinking that you don't want to feel tired and overwhelmed anymore and focusing on that thought, it may serve you better to focus your thoughts on wanting to feel vibrant, energetic, and able to breathe freely. Try it out for size and notice the difference.

So what does perfect health mean to you and how important is it? Each person will describe health differently depending on their own experiences, and likewise will place a different emphasis on it. If we fail to balance every aspect of our life, it is not unusual, or even surprising that our health is likely to be impacted.

I will use myself as an example once again. I have described several of the negative life events that affected me in my life, and how I never really dealt with them. In not dealing with them and placing a complete overemphasis on my work life and career, and on my relationships, which were far from healthy, neglecting to have any focus at all on fun and enjoyment, I eventually reached a breaking point. I got to a stage when I was so emotionally overwhelmed and completely overloaded with tasks that I just walked out of work one day, unable to hear anything but echoes coming from my staff as they called after me.

When I got home, I stripped off my clothes, climbed into bed, and slept for hours. I asked our nanny not to bring the children back for several hours. When I tried to get up, I couldn't even walk. It won't surprise you to hear that I of course went back to work the next day even though I was weak, shaky, and barely able to stand. I buried all of this and carried on, putting it down as a blip. There wasn't time to be ill!

Someone came into my life shortly afterwards who, having struggled with depression for over 10 years and been heavily medicated for it, was still having breakdowns. I helped him take ownership of his state instead of believing what the doctors had told him about taking more pills. He didn't have depression. It turns out he had chronic fatigue syndrome and could then work towards getting better. I remember thinking that if there was anything to learn from this relationship, it was that if I kept pushing myself I would end up just like him. Did I really want that?

I started to make huge changes in my life including selling my business. However, even that was to the detriment of my health. I had become so weak that despite never missing a day of work, I found myself unable to walk up the hill on my way home. Any time I got worked or stressed, I would have to sit down, such was the pain in my limbs. I couldn't even make it to the top floor of my house. I could still go to the gym and workout, but what was going on in my body was a very acute response to stress. My body was saying, "No more!" I had taken it so for granted that it was getting its own back.

A cardiologist diagnosed me as possibly having a condition called POTS. He advised me to read about it. The site was filled with stories about people who had led incredibly active lives only to suddenly be devastated and completely debilitated. I refused medication at that point and following a day of feeling very sorry for myself, I determined that there was no way I would allow any chronic illness to take over my life, and refused to own it. When I returned four months later, the cardiologist was surprised at how I had made a complete recovery and there was no sign of any illness.

EXERCISE PATH TO PERFECT HEALTH AND EXUBERANT ENERGY

Having perfect health and exuberant energy starts with defining for yourself what health is to you. The World Health Organization (WHO) defines health as "the state of complete physical, mental, and social well-being and not merely the absence of disease or infirmity."

One would expect health to be a balance between engaging in self-care, exercise, nutrition, feelings, and beliefs associated with vitality and positive thinking; how active you remain both physically and mentally; social relationships; and your support system.

I would love to introduce another iPEC foundation principle to you here.

"Pain is inevitable; suffering is optional."

What does this mean to you? For me it means that whatever we go through, we may well experience pain. It may be physical pain. It may be emotional pain because of something traumatic. It may be mental pain because we've cluttered our brains with so much that we can't think straight. However, even though we feel pain, we have a choice in whether or not, and how, we choose to suffer.

I can think of two of my patients who have gone through similar emotional traumas following divorce. They both experienced pain. One decided to let go of the anger and not let their former spouse's behavior impact them. They chose to move on with their lives and stood into their own power. I noticed the shift in them over the years as they started to present with more energy and vibrancy every time I saw them.

The other patient was obsessed by what happened. She held onto anger and resentment and the story was never-ending. It was shocking how in the space of the year, she aged, lost weight, started to lose her hair, and started to attract even more tragedies aside from the end of her marriage. One patient chose to suffer. The other did not. One chose to remain in a low energy frequency. The other chose to live life energetically.

As we have already discussed, such choices stem from our previous experiences and belief systems, but this is an example of how those choices can impact our health.

1- Pain vs Suffering

What pain have you experienced in your life and how have you suffered for it? List each painful experience and reflect on the effects that it may have led to. Allow what is deep inside you to emerge. Once it is down on paper you can start to recognize the patterns of your behavior, what blocks might be leading you to reenact those patterns, and then you'll be able to work on yourself to shift them by choosing new thoughts. This is not an easy task, but is well worth it.

What Painful Experience Has Happened For You?	What Impact Has It had On Your Life?

2- Try the **Peeling The Onion** exercise outlined in the previous chapter with a goal related to health in order to help you find a more sustainable motivator – an E-Motive.

3- Finding Your True Need

Download the worksheet for this from www.lightchangescoaching.com.

Draw three columns. In the first column, list all the things you don't want as they relate to health and aging. So it may be "I don't want to ache in the morning, I don't want to get wrinkly, I don't want to have pain," etc. Beside each of these statements, rewrite these statements in terms of what it is you DO want. In the case of not wanting to get wrinkly, a more positive statement would be that you want to have smooth, youthful skin. In the last column, write down what it is you believe that this desire will give you—why do you want it? How will it make you feel? Having smooth, youthful skin may make you feel young and vibrant, for example.

You may start to notice similarities in what you write down in this third column. This will give you a clue as to what need it is you have and how you are interpreting the fulfillment of this need being achieved. It will help you to identify your driving influences as they relate to health and aging, and focus your attention on achieving them.

Finding Your True Need

What Is It You Do Not Want?	Rephrase Into What You Do Want	What Need Will This Fulfill In You??

Summary for #Women Who Want More

I invite you to consider the following points related to leading a healthy, energetic life:

- What are your beliefs about health and how might they be limiting you?

- What are your beliefs about getting old and how might that be limiting you?

- What is it you worry most about in respect to your health?

- How much time do you spend worrying about your health?

- How many times do you say to yourself "I should" when it comes to engaging in a health-positive behavior?

- How might you seek support when trying to engage in health-positive behaviors?

- What might you consider asking a doctor the next time you are prescribed a medication?

- How might you take ownership of your health and seek to look after yourself first, before allowing others to do so?

- How might you incorporate gratitude for your health into your life?

- How might you consider incorporating mindfulness and meditation as a daily practice?

- How lonely do you feel if at all?

- Are there any patterns emerging that may give you a clue as to how are your thoughts and beliefs may be impacting your health?

Anything Is Possible!

You Just Have To Believe ...

#Insights

CHAPTER 9

MONEY:
I WANT MORE AND AM NOT ASHAMED
ABOUT IT

"It isn't enough for you to love money—it's also necessary that money should love you."
~ Kin Hubbard

What is having more money going to give you? How do you think you're going to feel when you clear your debt? How in control do you feel of your financial situation? How can you have more money?

I'd like you to visualize a scenario where you're walking along the road and notice someone holding a bundle of money. They are counting their money with a huge smile on their face. Then they hold the spread of notes up in the air in celebration. They start kissing the money and talking to it, all very publicly, inviting others to join them in this celebration.

What would you do in this situation? What would you do if that person made eye contact with you and held the money out to you to kiss? Would you join in? Would you think they were crazy and walk away? What thought comes up for you in that situation? Is it one of joy or one of disgust and disapproval at seeing someone delight in money that way? If you happened to be walking with a child, what would you tell them about the behavior you just witnessed?

Now picture another scenario. Once again, you're walking along the road and this time you notice someone is holding a baby. They are cradling the baby against their heart, touching its perfect little face, reaching down to kiss its forehead, and quite clearly whispering words of endearment. As they look up, they make eye contact with you, then smilingly turn the baby towards you, inviting you to join them in that love and delight.

What comes up for you in *this* situation? What would you do when that person made eye contact with you and showed you their baby? Would you smile back at them or perhaps step forward to admire the baby with them? Would you think they were crazy and walk away? What is the first thought you might be thinking when you walk past and witness the situation? Is it one of joy or is it one of disgust and disapproval at someone quite clearly loving their baby? If you happen to be walking with a child, what will you tell them about the behavior you just witnessed?

In the scenario with the baby, you would probably physically notice the baby responding to that love with its own smiles. By expressing love to the baby, a person is receiving love in return. The same applies to money. Even though we can't physically see the energy it gives off, it too will respond to you positively if you give off the same vibe. Conversely, why on earth would money choose to come to you if you are ashamed of it or think it might be dirty, and something that needs to be hidden away? If, in the case of somebody publicly loving money, thoughts of disapproval came up for you, you certainly are not alone. If you told the child with you that what you just witnessed was not right, again, you are not alone.

Your responses to these questions will give you a huge clue as to what your energetic response is to money, and whether you are going to attract or repel it. It is commonplace for us not to talk about money, even though the reality is most people would love to have more of it.

Money, just like everything else, is a form of energy. Think about how I introduced energy to you at the start of this book, stating the law in which energy cannot be created or destroyed. If we apply that to money, then I may have some, but use it to pay for groceries. The grocer then uses it to take his kids on a day out; the kids use it to pay for ice cream; the ice-cream vendor uses it to pay rent; the landlord uses it to reinvest; the investment fund manager uses it to generate more money; and so on and so on. Even when the money disappears from one person's hand, it continues to exist, but just in different forms, and with different people. Money, being a form of energy, flows abundantly. There is always enough for everybody.

Now that we have that clear, let's talk about where your balance lies with respect to finances and how you can get more money to flow to you.

Women in particular are exposed to more limiting beliefs when it comes to money. We grow up with stereotyping that a man is the provider of the household. Often our mothers stayed at home or only worked part-time, while men were the providers. We only need to look at society's divide in which men and women do not receive the same salaries for doing the same job to recognize the effect and impact this has on our belief systems growing up. If you were or are running a household, you may be the one managing the budget at home, whether or not you generated those funds. You may be given an allowance, in which case perhaps you don't feel completely in control of money. You may be single, in which case all the responsibility for your own care lies with you, and only you, and possibly for the care of your family. This may leave you feeling vulnerable, overwhelmed, driven with a sense of need, or a mixture.

One of my clients, who I'll call Tina, was married and worked part-time running her own business. Her husband earned more than her but they contributed to the household costs equally. Tina had grown up in an environment where money was scarce and had been taught to always make sure that you saved up for a rainy day. She was very organized with her finances and never overindulged. She would feel guilty about spending money on herself and even though there were savings in the bank, she never felt as if they were quite enough. Even though she worked hard, she always found generating money to be difficult. When she did earn a significant amount from her business, she would squirrel it away, and still feel as if there wasn't enough. She wouldn't take the opportunity to celebrate and would dread bills coming in. Tina's husband, on the other hand, would splash out, spend money frivolously—or so she felt—and had no savings. He believed that money would just come and there was no point in worrying about it.

In Tina's case it was quite clear that she didn't feel in control at all. She was approaching money from Level 1 energy where scarcity and lack were her primary thoughts. She would occasionally lift that energy level to Level 2, which would be one of anger and frustration with her husband, and with herself. The guilt in spending money, and the fear and dread of bills were all indicative of a catabolic energy state. She wanted more as she wanted control, but the energy she was emanating was not the type that was going to attract this to her. She was not in a state of flow in that she never wanted to spend money but only save it. She didn't have a sense of abundance. She couldn't share the same viewpoint as her husband and this in turn led to more catabolic energy.

The imbalance had an impact on Tina's relationship. She quite clearly hadn't set boundaries, part of which was communicating her needs to her husband, which would have helped her feel more in control. Her work was being affected in that her emphasis was much more on needing to make money rather than seeking fulfillment from the job itself. Life felt like a struggle.

We worked on her belief systems, firstly moving her to a place where she didn't react so catabolically to her husband's behavior. It won't surprise you that as their communication and relationship improved, he also shifted his spending habits to try to accommodate some of Tina's needs. We worked on her belief system as it related to money so she moved from a feeling of lack to one of gratitude and abundance, which are much higher energy levels. In shifting her energy, her thoughts, and her feelings, her actions and behavior also shifted. Her business started to thrive and she got more satisfaction. Life was no longer such a struggle and she resonated in energy states of gratitude and purpose. Tina was in control of her power.

The secret to having more money

Let's start with those limiting beliefs I mentioned earlier. Think about how we grew up and phrases that we have probably come across such as "money doesn't grow on trees," "money is evil, "I don't want to be like those rich people," "money spoils you," and "if you want to make money you have to work hard." Do any of these ring true for you? What's the first thought that might come up for you when you see somebody living in a big house or driving a fancy car? Is it one of envy, resentment, or celebration for them? All of these things should give you clues as to what beliefs may be holding you back.

If you have a belief system that money is scarce, the money will be scarce. If you believe that the only way to make money is to work incredibly hard, that's exactly what will happen. If you think that life is always a struggle, it will be. If you feel envy when you come across somebody who has money, this reveals your own sense of lack and that you are resonating at Level 1 because you may be thinking they are lucky ones and you are not, which means you are the victim. How common is it to buy a lottery ticket and in the same breath say, "I'd love to win the lottery but it'll never happen?" Then why are you even buying a ticket if you don't believe you have a chance?

Step One

Step one when it comes to bringing more money and abundance into your life is to identify what your limiting beliefs are and choose new beliefs. You might start by listing all your beliefs about money, and then rewrite them into more powerful ones. An example may be a belief that "you have to work incredibly hard in order to earn money." A more empowering new belief would be "money is abundant and comes to me easily." You might change "money doesn't grow on trees" to "money is everywhere; it is available to everyone from all sources." You could also state affirmations such as "I love money," "money is my friend," "I feel good about receiving money."

Step Two

Step two is the need to feel deserving of money. This essentially means working on forgiving and loving yourself so that you feel worthy of receiving money in the same way as you need to feel you are worthy of receiving love. I recall a conversation with one of my clients where she had been given the opportunity to go on a world cruise at no cost to herself. My client kept repeating, "I can't believe this has happened to me!" She just kept repeating it over and over, and even though she wanted to accept, was having great difficulty in doing so. She didn't feel worthy or deserving of such a gift. I remember saying to her, "You're sounding as if it's a bad thing by saying this happened 'to' you! Why don't you think that this may have happened *for* you and you are fully deserving of it?" That is a far more empowering thought.

It's all very well having people tell us that we deserve something, but the belief must come from within us. I know in my own past experience when someone gave me a gift, or bought me dinner, the first thing I wanted to do was give them something in return. What I should have been doing was accepting the gift gracefully and joyously, rather than overwhelmingly wanting to make sure I gave them something back, which was indicative of having a deep sense of unworthiness. The same applies to compliments: a gift is a compliment. How do you receive it? I used to feel embarrassed and immediately returned a present. Now, when my partner says how lucky he is to have me in his life and wonders what on earth he did to deserve me, I respond, "Yes, you are lucky, and you must have asked for me, so here I am!"

Why do you want to have money? If your only answer is so that you can help others, then essentially you are radiating out an energy that suggests you yourself are not worthy of having it and must only pass it on. That may seem harsh because you are quite clearly incredibly generous and full of love, but just like how you need to put the mask on yourself in an airplane before you put it on your children, you need to love yourself and give to yourself before giving to others.

Step Three

Step three is to free up some space. If you are filled with thoughts and feelings of resentment towards those who do have money, then you are blocking your own flow. If you sit in judgment on how others spend their money, then you are using up your energy on that (a catabolic energy state), where it would be better used on one of joy, love, and gratitude (anabolic energy states). If you dread your bills, and open them up with fear and trepidation, then you are clogging yourself up with the energy of fear. You need to release these in order to create space and allow abundance and the energy of wealth to flow through you. You could try to love your bills by opening up the credit card statement and recalling all the joy you felt from buying things; you could think how the electricity provides a comfortable home, or the phone allows you to connect with people, and consider how grateful you are for that, rather than being resentful of the piece of paper that asks you to pay for it all.

You can take this even further to material things. Think about the kitchen cupboards that haven't been cleaned out for a while, or the filing cabinet that has gathered dust, or the staleness of the house when you come back after a long holiday and the windows and doors haven't been opened. How good does it feel when you empty out your wardrobes and give away old clothes to charity? What's the natural thing that happens when you have space in your closet? I know mine gets filled up again with new clothes and new shoes! The same applies to allowing wealth to come into your life. You need to make space. Giving away old toys that no longer serve your household but could be a benefit to somebody else is a way of passing on wealth. Giving away what you no longer need (both emotional and physical) creates space for something else to fill that vacuum.

Step Four

Once you've rid yourself of all the catabolic energy within you and have created space, step four is to rejoice, allow, and give gratitude. You need to open your arms up to receiving, feel the expansion of energy and abundance within you, and truly believe that it is limitless. There is enough for everybody. Think about standing on a beach and looking out at the ocean. You may see the horizon but you know that beyond that, there is more water. Try to think of money in the same way—you know it is there even if you can't see it. There's no need to limit it just because it's not yet tangible. Visualization can really help engage in these feelings of freedom and abundance.

It's very easy to get fixated on the "how." *How* can I get more money? *How* much more money can I make in this job? You need to let go of that attachment. These are limiting thoughts and by giving out energy that you only want to receive money in a certain way, which may mean you think it can only happen through work, for example, then there is no way it can happen any other way because your energy will not allow it. Celebrating every small achievement will bring you more. If you're grateful for receiving even a small amount, it will start to lift your energy and reinforce your beliefs of what is possible and in turn you will create more to be grateful for in your reality. It might mean that you start off with £100 more a month, but by rejoicing and giving gratitude for just that, your energy will lift and you will radiate energy and engage in behaviors that continue to attract even more into your life.

The Four Gets™

I call these steps *The Four Gets™*. They can be applied to any aspect of your life:

1- **Get Out** – get the limiting beliefs out of your head

2- **Get Loving** – start loving yourself and feeling worthy

3- **Get Rid** – of resentment, fear, judgment, and clutter

4- **Get Going** – with actions to receive, allow, appreciate, and celebrate

The law of attraction outlines three steps. It states that you need to Ask, Believe, and Receive. We've covered these points already in that you need to visualize and ask for what you want without being attached to the outcome or the how. You need to truly believe that it's going to happen which you can do by releasing the limiting beliefs and energy blocks and clearing clutter. And then you need to be ready to receive by allowing it to happen, coming from a place of desire rather than desperate need, and give gratitude as if you really believe that it has already happened. You then need to congratulate yourself and celebrate.

Derek Rydall, in his book *The Abundance Project*, describes a similar approach with what he calls the Seven Gives. He talks about the need to:

○ Give Forth by sharing your time, talent, and treasure

○ Give Away by circulating what you no longer need or use

○ Give Up by releasing habits, judgments, criticisms, and complaints

- ○ Give In by letting go of the resistance and surrendering

- ○ For-Giving by freeing yourself from those emotional blocks

- ○ Give To yourself by giving to yourself what you seek from others

- ○ Give Thanks for what you appreciate

EXERCISE PATH TO CREATING MORE FINANCIAL FULFILMENT

1- Core Beliefs

We've talked already about exercises you can do to uncover your limiting beliefs so it's a good idea to write those down and beside them write down new empowering beliefs to override them, as well as positive affirmations in alignment with those new beliefs. Revisit the Core-Beliefs exercise in chapter 5, reapplying it as it relates to your beliefs about money.

Core belief about money	
Who taught me this?	
Do I still want it?	
What's a new belief to replace it?	

Core belief about money	
Who taught me this?	
Do I still want it?	
What's a new belief to replace it?	

2- Abundance Tool

We've also talked about visualization. I have prepared a guided meditation for you which you can download from www.lightchangescoaching.com. I talk you through The Four Gets™ process. I will help you to form a vision of what abundance looks like to you, uncover what you believe it is that may be blocking you, and really engage in the feelings and beliefs of having what it is you want as well as the essential component of gratitude. If money and abundance are a big focus for you, then I would recommend listening to this meditation on a daily basis for at least two weeks with a view to shifting your energy in that direction.

3- £100 Virtual Shopping Spree

The next exercise can be a lot of fun and very empowering. You can change the name to suit whatever currency you deal in. The first thing to do is to carry around £100 (or $100 if that's your currency) in your purse or wallet. You need to remember that it's there. Then, whenever you see something that you might want to buy with that £100, say to yourself in your head, "I can buy that but I choose not to." You can shop online and find lots of things that you think you might want but don't need (shoes in my case!!!) and, knowing that you have the £100 in your purse, of course you can buy them, but choose not to.

Do that for a month. It will start to shift your energy into one of abundance because you are stepping into the power of deservedness and possibility and the power of making your own choices and decisions. I've done this exercise with my kids before and now I find them almost habitually saying, "We could buy that but we choose not to," as opposed to "we can't afford to," which would be coming from a place of lack. It's incredibly empowering and a lot of fun!

4- Abundance And Money-Flow Journal

Keep an abundance and money-flow journal. Each day, list the money you are receiving, both in terms of real money and also savings you may have made, and the money that you have chosen to give away be it in the form of gifts, charitable contributions, an investment in your home, business, or yourself, such as a holiday. Essentially you want to be able to see the benefits of having given the money away. As you reflect on each month's income, give gratitude for receiving that money and the sources from which it came. At the bottom of each page write a powerful affirmation which might be something along the lines of "I am so grateful and deserving of the ease with which money flows to me and through me." It's worth using different affirmations on different days and I'm sure you'll be guided to come up with different things depending on your mood or energetic resonance. Notice any feelings that might arise as you are making entries in the journal as that may give you clues to whether or not you still have any limiting beliefs. Also notice the shift of what happens over time as you start to invite the flow of abundance into your life.

Summary for #Women Who Want More

I invite you to consider the following points:

- Money is an energy and we need to allow it to flow through us

- What do you believe money to be truly for?

- When does money energize you? When does it drain you?

- How do you feel about having tremendous wealth?

- What is it you think money will give you? The answer to that question is probably what you're truly seeking

- Feelings of lack, scarcity, guilt, anger, and judgment are catabolic energy states which do not serve us in attracting abundance into our lives

- Consider *The Four Gets*™ as a means of clearing out catabolic energy and shifting into an anabolic energy state

- Nothing is in isolation—if we have an imbalance where focus lies purely on monetary concerns, then other aspects of our lives may be affected

- The balance within issues to do with personal finance can be made up of our income, expenses, budgeting, investments, organization, financial planning, our legacy and estate, and our abundance consciousness

- There is always enough for everybody

*"The source of all abundance is not outside you.
It is part of who you are."*

~ Eckhart Tolle

#Insights

CHAPTER 10

MAKING IT FUN
AND FINDING THE TIME!!!!

"Time is more valuable than money. You can get more money, but you cannot get more time."
~ Jim Rohn

How much fun are you having in your life? Are you relying on other people to create the fun for you? How busy are you doing other things that you can't make time for fun? How overwhelmed do you feel by lack of time?

When it comes to our priorities, particularly for women in a Western society, fun tends to be very low on the list. We are so busy juggling our careers, families, and relationships, that specifically making time for fun on a daily basis might not even enter our thought process. Having fun is often something you feel you have to do in isolation. This might mean taking a vacation, going on a weekend retreat, going out to dinner or drinks, or engaging in a cultural activity. We isolate the time between fun and the rest of our lives as opposed to integrating it. If you really do run out of time having been to work, done the laundry, cooked dinner, helped the kids with homework, gone to the gym, and then are thoroughly exhausted, that plan you may have had for fun and relaxation goes out the window. It becomes one of those "I'll get to it" tasks, and if we try to force the issue, we are usually too distracted to be fully present and in the moment, therefore failing to experience the true sense of enjoyment. The sense of being *in*-joy (en-joy).

Think about those times when you are going to a party, New Year's Eve being a prime example. The expectation in those situations is so high that you're going to be having fun that it is frequently a letdown. Conversely, think of those spontaneous occasions where a friend may have unexpectedly called round for tea, or you've stayed out later than expected, or have found yourself doing something unplanned. You may well find that when you reflect on that, the latter may have been more enjoyable. The latter is something that may have allowed you to feel freedom because it wasn't in the plan

Joy often comes from the unexpected. Think about children and how they seek to have joy in every moment of their lives. Everything is a potential adventure to them. They don't know everything that's going to happen that day and so look at the world from a point of curiosity and engagement. They haven't yet been weighed down with responsibilities and "musts" and "shoulds." They haven't yet been weighed down by fears that prevent them from being present and in the moment. They expect the unexpected and relish in what that can bring, rather than being paralyzed by it.

How exciting could life be if you were willing to experience that sense of fun and enjoyment in every aspect of your life and throughout your day, as opposed to needing to compartmentalize it into a time slot that takes away the spontaneity and gets sacrificed for other things?

When I first signed up with a coach a few years ago, she gave me an assignment based on what I wanted to be doing in a year's time. I recall writing down that I wanted to be having fun! I was doing very little aside from working incredibly hard, slotting in time for regular exercise, and looking after my kids. I was still going on holiday, traveling the world for work, and catching up with friends, so what was the problem? You would have thought that with all that going on, I should be able to find some opportunities for fun. But my energy was such that I wasn't able to see the opportunities for fun in traveling to different countries. I wasn't able to see the opportunities for fun in just talking with my children or in my everyday work life. I was too busy to notice. Too busy to be present.

So here we go again: it all comes down to where your energy lies. As for finding time; that, frankly, was inconceivable. A friend of mine tried to advise me to organize my diary so that I could identify exactly how much time I was spending treating patients, traveling, or going to meetings and so on. The idea was that it would get things out of my head to help declutter me and make me feel less stressed because I would have a visual of the time available to me. Such was my stress level at the time that I was completely overwhelmed with that task— one that was supposed to help me with time! I didn't have time to make time! Even making appointments with my coach, who was going to help me, was a stress and imposition on my available time!

Eventually I shifted my energy from one of lack, which we've talked about being Level 1 and catabolic, to one of abundance, which is Level 6 and highly anabolic. I went from believing that there was no time for anything and feeling undeserving to one of enjoyment, love, gratitude, purpose, and belief that time was available to me very readily, and that fun was not something I needed, but something I deserved. This isn't something that happens overnight, but by gradually shifting my mindset, and taking baby steps, I was able to move towards the larger goal. I had to apply the same principles of *The Four Gets*™ that I described in the last chapter, and if I'm honest, I don't think it was really a conscious thing, but in carrying out that process, and setting the initial intention, and then taking the baby steps to allowing it to happen, it truly did.

I'll talk more about that healing journey to living a truly joyous and fulfilled life in the next chapter, but I will share with you now that one thing I did was reengage with my inner child. I've already talked about how children view each day with adventure and curiosity, and approach things with playfulness. There had always been that side to me, but I had buried it. I reengaged with the innocence and shed my inhibitions.

I started to integrate fun into my working life. I would take time to engage with my staff rather than burying myself at my desk catching up on emails at lunchtime. I had always laughed and joked with my patients, but there was no time to do it with my staff. Strangely, I still managed to get all the tasks done. I found purpose and fulfillment once again through the leadership that we talked about in the earlier chapters. That meant that by going to work and being present, I was experiencing enjoyment. By *choosing* to go to work with an open mind and a sense of anticipation and excitement, as opposed to a feeling of dread and fear of what the day might hold, I was engaging in that childlike energy and in turn attracting the same high energy back to myself.

I adopted a "what's the worst that could happen?" approach to activities that I never considered before. The image this brings to my mind is my seven-year-old parading around naked on a sailing boat around the Greek islands. Did he care that he was naked? No! He felt free! Everyone else had a problem with it—not him! While I may not have paraded around naked on a sailboat for all to see, I have done some pretty crazy things like going to a naked restaurant! I didn't stop laughing about that experience for over a week and if we ever meet I'll happily tell you about how the logistics worked! For now, I will confirm that the lighting was tasteful.

I've run into the freezing sea in Brighton in the month of November with nothing but the moonlight to show the way; I have danced on a beach with a friend where I created a silent disco, and not cared that anybody might wonder what I was doing. And guess what? Just like with gratitude, because I had started resonating an energy of *en-joyment*, even more fun and enjoyment came into my life. I have walked along the Great Wall of China, climbed to the top of Sydney Harbor bridge, drunk champagne with Her Majesty the Queen, and screamed in delight with my arms outstretched at the top of mountains. Somehow there was time for it all ...

Another factor to consider is who you are surrounding yourself with. How do you feel when you are with them? If they are highly energetic, then the chances are you will feel the same around them. If on the other hand you feel drained, then this is a clue to where their energy charge lies, and the effect it is having on you. This can certainly impact your fun and enjoyment. If you are in a partnership and the other person can never come up with ideas for fun, or then takes part in your ideas, but without much enthusiasm, then that is going to impact your experience. Also remember that what is fun for one is not necessarily fun for the other, so beware of always trying to please the other person by sacrificing yourself. Think high energy; think win-win, rather than low energy, which would be "you win, I lose," or "I win, you lose."

The secret to finding time and having fun

Let me share another one of iPECs foundation principles:

"Life is a perfect adventure; a game that cannot be won or lost, only played."

The first step is to shift your mindset to view everything with curiosity, adventure, and opportunity, and yet not be fixated on how it's going to turn out. That gives you power and freedom. You release the control. You may not know how it's going to turn out or what's around the corner, but it doesn't matter—as long as you play the game. As long as you are present and in the moment.

How can you do it? Well, practicing mindfulness helps tremendously. Meditation to clear your head from distractions is another. If we go back to multitasking, then combining either of those with an activity you find fun can be a really effective way of managing your time. You might choose to engage in mindful walking. You could go dancing and meditate at the same time. You may have heard of 5Rhythms—developed by Gabrielle Roth, she describes it as a way of meditating and dancing in the same breath. You can engage your creative side with mindfulness coloring books. Simply taking a few breaths and centering yourself before any task can help you settle and become present.

Once you are in the moment, looking for fun, you are much more likely to find it. Think of frantically looking for your credit card in your purse. If it's not where you expect, you start to panic and search even more frantically. You may find it later, when you are much calmer, in a pocket you had looked in before, but such was your state of mind that you didn't see it, even though it was right in front of you.

Affirmations at the start of your day will also help set the energetic tone for the day. If you start your day saying, "I know today is going to be stressful," or "Today is going to a nightmare!" then you have set your energy to expect just that, and that is what you will see and experience. An alternative viewpoint could be "my eyes and mind are open to all opportunities for adventure today and I will be present to see and experience them," or "no matter what the day throws at me, I can cope and have fun with it!" You may not feel it, but just like with any physical exercise where repeated training is the key, the more you say it, the stronger your belief will become.

It can feel scary stepping into the unknown. If that is the case, what is it that is scaring you? Go deeper until you find out. Only then can you deal with it so it doesn't seem so scary anymore. Think about being a child afraid of the dark; the dressing gown hanging on the back of the door looks like a monster. When the light comes on, you realize it was just a dressing gown and nothing to fear after all. In just the same way that you can unhook the dressing gown and get rid of it, you can do the same with your fears—but you have to take action.

The next thing to consider is how guilty you feel in taking time to go out and have fun. How unproductive do you feel because of it? Your responses to these questions will reveal if you are feeling undeserving of having fun—in which case you need to prescribe yourself some self-love and forgiveness. The answers to these questions will also tell you about where your priorities lie. If you are asking for more fun and enjoyment and then feeling like it has wasted your time and you didn't have a chance to complete an assignment or get the housework done, then there is a disconnect between your inner and outer desires. The inner desires are the energy you are resonating, and the outer desires are what you are asking for out loud.

I'll use an example of a colleague. I'll call her Emily. Emily had her own business which had gone from strength to strength, so much so that she was in high demand and feeling overwhelmed, not having enough time to meet the demands of her clients. She had a waiting list and where she had previously had days off, they were now becoming few and far between. While there was now plenty of money and business success, she was struggling to find time to have fun. What use was money if she couldn't enjoy it? Yes, she was helping people, which made her feel good, but it was starting to drain her. She also wasn't in a relationship, and wanted to meet someone and hopefully have children. How was she supposed to find time for that if she was working 24-7? I'm sure by now you'll recognize the energetic imbalance where one aspect of life suffers due to an over-focus of energy in another area. Let's break this down a little further.

First, Emily wanted time for a relationship, and voiced it, but still filled her diary with appointments. Her actions were not in sync with her desires. There was also a boundaries issue here in that she was allowing clients to move into her personal time. Those clients wouldn't have known that she didn't usually book appointments past 7 p.m. and that she was making an exception unless she told them, which she didn't. Then she harbored resentment. She felt guilt in taking time out for vacation because she thought she would be letting clients down and also believed she would be even more overwhelmed when she came back to work. These fears showed an inner lack of deserving and being too distracted to be present and enjoy the time on vacation—already focusing on what she might face upon her return.

Then let's add into the mix the deeper fear that she might make the time in her diary, but then what if she didn't meet anyone? It was easier to tell herself that the reason she wasn't in a relationship was because she didn't have time.

This whole situation on the surface seemed like one of time management, when in fact it was so much more energetically charged. Charged with catabolic energy—lack of control, guilt, fear, and limiting beliefs.

If all we had done was give Emily a strategy to block off time like my friend tried with me, it never would have worked long-term. She had to *get out* of the limiting belief mindset, *get loving* herself, honor her values, honor her boundaries, honor her priorities, and *get rid* of resentment, fear, and clutter, all before we could *get going* on the action steps. Some of these included blocking out time specifically for fun just like she did with appointments with clients so that she couldn't double-book herself; she color-coded her diary to get a visual on how much time she was allocating for fun and enjoyment. She celebrated every time she turned down additional work that would have impacted her fun time and started to view time as abundant. She gave gratitude for all the experiences of fun in her life. By taking control, Emily resonated from a higher energy frequency and stepped into her power.

Where do your priorities lie when it comes to having fun and enjoyment? What is it you think it will give you? It may be you believe it will improve your health, or help you to experience your kids growing up more, or like in the last example, open up space for a relationship. Once you reveal the underlying desire behind the label of fun and enjoyment, then this becomes a deeper, more heartfelt motivator. You can apply the Peeling The Onion exercise to this beautifully, and it will help to keep you on track, particularly in a busy life where you have so many priorities. Setting boundaries, honoring them, and ensuring others also honor them is paramount when it comes to succeeding in sticking to priorities.

It's workout time! How much fun is this going to be?!!!

EXERCISE PATH TO FITTING IN TIME FOR FUN

1- Put Fun To Paper

List all the things that you might like to do for fun. Fun is relative, with what is fun for one person not necessarily being the case for everyone. When you make this list, try your best not to limit it by thinking about the "how." If you want to try sky-diving and think you'll never afford it, then you are limiting the possibility right there.

2- Adding Seasoning To My Life

List all the aspects of your life in one column—work/career, relationships, health, making money, parenting, personal development, spirituality. In each section, write down how you might engage in fun within that field. I've told you about how at home we fill our family gratitude jar. When it's full, we then go out in the garden and burn all the pieces of paper and dance around the garden releasing all the ashes into the universe. As the ashes sink down into the soil, we also view it as planting the seeds for growth. This is just one way I integrate fun into spirituality and parenting. You might decide to bake cookies with your child, and you might also choose to sell them at a fundraiser. That might then cover a means of having fun in the area of parenting/family, money and spirituality. Yet more multitasking!! Do I hear a woo-hoo?!!! Download the worksheet from www.lightchangescoaching.com.

Aspects Of My Life	How I Can Season It With Fun

3- Engage Your Inner Child

List ways in which you might be able to engage your inner child. If you have children then they may well be an inspiration for this and can offer up some ideas, I'm sure. It may even be something you choose to do together. We have a Sunday ritual once a month where the kids choose to have anything they want for breakfast. Ice cream is a fairly regular choice. I just go with it, let go of the control, and enjoy the chance to be inappropriately silly. A word of warning here though—I'd avoid adding jelly beans to the mix: they lose their chewiness when they get too cold!

Ways I may be able to engage my inner child:

4- Finding More Time

List the Big A **A**genda items in your life—meaning the things that only you can do. Then list the Little A **a**genda items, where '**a**' is things that others might be able to do for you. Review your list—is everything in the '**A**' list nonnegotiable? If there is anything that could be negotiated, consider that it may be possible to move it into the '**a**' list, and vice versa. To offer an example here—spending quality time with my kids is a nonnegotiable, so it goes in the 'A' list. Washing and ironing, which while it serves my kids, also takes time away from them, goes in the '**a**' list and I have a housekeeper who comes in to do it for me.

When you start thinking about this and open your mind up to the possibilities, it's very empowering. A classic example is related to work. I could spend another two hours after work typing up patient reports, or I could dictate those in 20 minutes, pay to have them transcribed and have more time of other things. Just something to consider if you start voicing excuses. Open your mind to possibility. Once you make a decision to change, consider engaging in the deeper motivation and write it down somewhere you can see it to keep you on track to maintain the behavior change and let go of the reins.

Finding More Time

The 'A' Items Non-Negotiable Things Only You Can Do	The 'a' Items Things That You May Be Able To Delegate After All To Free Up Time

"Dance like no one is watching,
Live like you'll never be hurt
Sing like no one is listening
Live like it's heaven on earth."

~ William Purkey

Summary for #Women Who Want More

I'd invite you to consider the following as they relate to fun, enjoyment, and time:

- How can you integrate fun into your daily life?

- Practicing mindfulness allows you to be present

- Meditation clears space for you to be present

- Overcoming fears allows you to be curious and engage in adventure

- Engage your inner child

- Start your day with affirmations of positivity and abundance

- Give up control every now and again and just surrender to what comes

- Consider delegating tasks

- Set boundaries and priorities, and honor them

- Are your behavior and actions in line with your inner desires?

#Insights

CHAPTER 11

YES – I CAN!!!

"Experience is not what happens to you; it's what you do with what happens to you."
~ Aldous Huxley

We've gone very deep in this book. I have shared with you thoughts, stories, and strategies, and asked you some challenging questions.

SO NOW IT'S TIME TO LIGHTEN THE MOOD!

I'd love you to reenergize so that you can come back and focus!

Your mission—should you choose to accept it—is one of two. Remember: there is *always* a choice!

1- Choose your favorite high-energy song—the one that would always be a top choice if you were asking a DJ to play it for you. Put it on loud, and go dance. *Dance* around your home like no one is watching you; *sing* as loud as you can, like no one can hear you. If you're on a train or surrounded by people where you can't make noise or dance—then put on your headphones and dance and sing in your head. No one else needs to know what you're doing. Just let loose!

2- The other option, equally effective, so it's purely personal preference, is to download the five-minute centering exercise if you haven't done so already from www.lightchangescoaching.com and listen to it. Then come back.

The Secret of Energetic Balance

In this book we have talked a lot about how there is no good or bad energy. How there is catabolic and anabolic and how either may show up in your thoughts, feelings, and behaviors. I've shown you examples of how when that energy is not balanced in all aspects of your life, other parts can suffer as a consequence.

I'd like you to imagine a flower with petals surrounding it. You are that flower and stand in the center of it. Each of those petals represents an aspect of your life. Your relationships, both social and intimate; your family; career or professional life; health; financial life; fun and enjoyment; and your personal development and spiritual life, whatever that means to you, which we discussed at the start of this book. While standing in the center of the flower, everything is in balance. That doesn't necessarily mean all is equal—the petals of your flower may be different sizes, but while you are standing in the middle, it's not going anywhere. It is present.

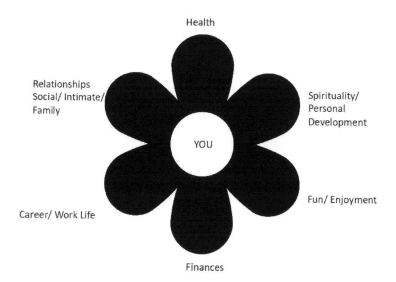

If you step from the center of the flower onto one of those petals, it may tip a little, but won't collapse completely as you haven't strayed too far from the center. If it's one of the bigger petals, it can withstand more before it starts to tip. If you keep walking to the edge of the petal, however, eventually it will reach critical mass and start to tip.

In most cases, it won't collapse completely, so there is time to crawl back towards the center. You might hang there for a while, then test your footing again on another petal, and the same thing may happen. You may reach a crisis and head back in. This may happen several times. Depending on how strong the stalk is, eventually it will not only bend, but will snap.

When the stalk is bending, the water can still make its way into the flower to feed it, though the route is slightly more diverted and it may take a bit longer. But if the stalk snaps, the water can't get around those kinks. The channels will be blocked and the flower will wither. Not only that, but in its collapse, the stalk might have leaned so heavily on the flowers next to it that they can't support the weight anymore and they get pushed down also.

I'm sure you can see where we are going with this. You are the flower, standing proud in all your glory with a strong stalk, surrounded by a social network of other flowers—other people. Energy runs through you just like the water running up the stalk, and it spreads out into the petals. The more weight and the further you step out onto one petal, the more energy needs to go there to keep it up. Think about the phrases we commonly use—"I put all my energy into that task"; "I put all my energy into that relationship!" Ultimately it can be to the detriment of the surrounding petals—the other aspects of your life, and then eventually to the detriment of the whole flower—which is you, and possibly the surrounding flowers, which represent the other people around you.

Now I'm not saying you have to hang out in the center of the flower all the time. Where would the fun be in that if you always had the same view? Of course there will be times in your life when your focus is weighted in one direction more than others. Times in your life you devote more attention to your relationships, your home life, your kids, your work. The trick is not to step out so far away that the other areas cry out and because they can't be heard, they kick up a fuss so that you start listening and pay attention to them. Think about your own life where you may have experienced such a wake-up call.

Have you ever considered that you can also change the view by rotating around the middle portion of the flower without needing to step onto the petals? Standing on any part of that center—it doesn't have to be bang in the center—will keep you in balance. The energy will be able to flow through you and distribute outward.

That is what energetic balance means. That is the secret.

What my balance looks like

Thank you for allowing me to share so much of my story with you. I have shared with you my journey, the crises I have experienced, the clear imbalance I had, the bends in the stalk, and my last wake-up call of being diagnosed with a chronic illness. That was when I eventually stepped fully back to the middle of my flower.

How did I do it?

I started my healing. I started practicing all the things I have discussed with you in this book. I cried for a whole month after having a Reiki healing session, such was the release of energy that I had trapped in me. I started to stand in my own power. Even though I had hired a coach a few years earlier, it wasn't the type of coaching I have been talking about. We had focused primarily on shifting my 'what' rather than my "who," so up until then, I hadn't really changed and kept repeating old patterns.

I started to practice mindfulness, meditation, being open about my spirituality, and showing it to everybody instead of just a select few. I spent time with a shaman who helped me to heal from the patterns of abusive and destructive behavior and taught me about the luminous energy field surrounding our bodies which holds all of our history in it and affects us physically. I trained in Rahanni healing which is a fifth-dimensional healing based on energy. I practiced healing on myself daily. I joined a spiritual circle in order to develop my intuitive skills and to actually speak with my guides rather than ignoring them. The more I did, the more energy I felt and the more I was guided to further opportunities for healing.

I made the decision to sell my business, recognizing that I was and would always still be a leader. I controlled my work life instead of letting it control me. The same applied to food and my health. I reprioritized my life, concentrating more on my kids, my health, and fun. I let go of the things and people that were making me unhappy, and the things I couldn't let go of, I chose to no longer react to in the same destructive way. I identified what was important to me in a relationship, but let go of the need for one. When I was ready, the right one came into my life. One where I now have boundaries and we grow together. One that is balanced.

I expressed gratitude every day. I recognized that while I had spent years rising to the heights of my profession and helping people, there was more to life than just that and I had a greater purpose. I asked for help in finding that, and was guided to become a coach. Not just any coach—in fact, when I was accepted in a different course and went to pay, my card payment wouldn't go through—such is the power of the universe. Then I found iPEC and trained to be a core-energy™ coach, and felt compelled to write this book to share with you the significance of energy balance. I hope that my story can inspire you to find it too.

Everyone now describes me as having vibrant energy because I now show up the same way to all people in my life. It radiates out of me. I am present. I recognize that not all of this will resonate with you and it doesn't have to, but this is just an example about how in listening to myself and to my higher self or higher coach or whatever you choose to call it, I was finally able to step into my new life. A life where I DO HAVE IT ALL! I have fulfillment, *and* I have balance.

The Journey Doesn't End Here ...

The journey doesn't end here; it *starts* here!

I'm sure by reading this book, you have gained insights into your own life and I hope you feel inspired to apply what you have learned. Insights on their own are not enough. Without actions and a willingness to do the work, nothing will change for you. You will remain stuck, repeating the same cycles over and over.

I asked you at the start of this book, what it is you want in your life? Start there, and use the exercises in this book to help propel you forward into action. Find your deep core motivators that will help drive you to sustain the changes you want to make and lead a purposeful life. Remember, you can download the exercises and meditations from www.lightchangescoaching.com and may choose to work on them systematically, or when needed. However, the daily centering exercise will prove invaluable to your journey and is a great starting point.

Practice **THE FOUR GETS™** to get what it is you want

1- **Get Out** – get the limiting beliefs out of your head

2- **Get Loving** – start loving yourself, feeling worthy, honoring boundaries

3- **Get Rid** – of resentment, fear, judgment, and physical and mental clutter

4- **Get Going** – with actions to receive, allow, appreciate, and celebrate

It will help get you far!

If you need help, then please ask for it. You don't have to do this alone. Tell your friends, your family, your work colleagues, so they can all share in the journey, and you can support each other. Hiring a coach can help more in that is takes something generalized like a book to something so much more personalized to you and your life and circumstances.. More information about coaching, courses, and suggested further reading is on my website. Even if we are not a fit or I can't help you directly, I may be able to direct you to someone who can. Or just get in touch for the hell of it—I love to connect with people.

If you are curious to know where your energy resonates in each aspect of your life or as it relates to the desire to do certain tasks, then there is an assessment you can take called the Energy Leadership Index (ELI), after which you will need to be debriefed by an ELI master practitioner (ELI-MP). This assessment can be for one individual or a whole company. Again, further details are available on my website.

And Finally ...

I'm not suggesting that you follow my path and do the same things I did. You are your own person and need to make your own path. To share another iPEC foundation principle with you:

"Each person's journey is as unique and valuable as the others."

You need to step into your own power. In so doing, next time someone asks you, "Can you really have everything you want in life? Can you really have it all?"

You'll answer, "YES—I CAN!"

"How? What's the secret?"

"The answer lies within you!"